RATIONING HEALTH CARE IN AMERICA

Rationing Health Care in America:

Perceptions and Principles of Justice

LARRY R. CHURCHILL

University of Notre Dame Press
Notre Dame, Indiana

The Parable of the American is from
The Pursuit of Loneliness, rev. ed., by Philip Slater
Copyright © 1970, 1976 by Philip E. Slater
Reprinted by permission of Beacon Press.

Library of Congress Cataloging in Publication Data

Churchill, Larry R., 1945–
    Rationing health care in America.

    Bibliography: p.
    Includes index.
    1. Medical care—United States—Utilization.
2. Medical ethics—United States. 3. Social
medicine—United States. I. Title. [DNLM:
1. Health Policy—United States. 2. Health
Services Accessibility—United States. 3. Human
Rights. 4. Philosophy, Medical. W 61 C563r]
    RA410.7.C48   1987   362.1'0973   86-40582
    ISBN 0-268-01630-5

FOR SANDE

All people of broad, strong sense have an instinctive repugnance to the men of maxims; because such people early discern that the mysterious complexity of our life is not to be embraced by maxims, and that to lace ourselves up in formulas of that sort is to repress all the divine promptings and inspirations that spring from growing insight and sympathy. And the man of maxims is the popular representative of the minds that are guided in their moral judgment solely by general rules, thinking that these will lead them to justice by a ready-made patent method, without the trouble of exerting patience, discrimination, impartiality, without any care to assure themselves whether they have the insight that comes from a hardly-earned estimate of temptation, or from a life vivid and intense enough to have created a wide fellow-feeling with all that is human.

George Eliot, *The Mill on the Floss* (1860)

Contents

Acknowledgments

Every individual work presupposes a convivial community which nurtures and supports it. This book is no exception. The debts I have incurred in writing it are large.

Glenn Wilson, Chair of the Department of Social and Administrative Medicine at UNC, and Stuart Bondurant, Dean of the UNC School of Medicine, generously supported a sabbatical leave during the Summer and Fall of 1985. It was during this time that most of the writing was done.

Many colleagues and friends have discussed with me the ideas presented here, critically read part or all of the manuscript, or otherwise stimulated me to better formulations. Among these are James Childress, Stanley Hauerwas, Gail Henderson, Nancy King, William McGaghie, Glenn Pickard, Pam Silberman, José Simán, Harmon Smith, Ruel Tyson, Richard Vance, and Glenn Wilson. I am grateful for their many contributions, though I sometimes stubbornly refused to follow their advice. I owe Case Study 2 to Glenn Pickard, my teaching partner with house officers in the Department of Medicine. I thank Jean Oliver, once again, for her skill and patience as a typist.

I am particularly indebted to Harmon Smith, my co-author in a previous work, *Professional Ethics and Primary Care Medicine*. A good deal of the intellectual momentum for this essay came from that collaboration.

While all the words were written in Chapel Hill, this book took its definitive shape during three successive weeks in Europe: the first in Helsinki at the IX Social Sciences and Medicine Conference, the next at the King's Fund College in London, and the last at a Hastings Center Conference at

Queen's College, Oxford. At each location I found stimulating conversation partners and I want to acknowledge the organizations which sponsored these conferences and visits.

Finally, to Sande, Shelley, and Blair, who are sources of great joy for me, I offer special thanks. Much of what I know about the human situation that makes me hopeful I owe to them.

Introduction

Ten years ago Dr. Howard Hiatt, then Dean of the Harvard School of Public Health, published an article in the *New England Journal of Medicine* asking whose responsibility it is to protect the medical commons.[1] Hiatt cited rising medical costs, ineffective procedures, and traditions of individual freedom as all contributing to the problem of an increasingly diminished and endangered commons of health resources. The article was politely received but drew little critical notice. The reason was not that the issue was unimportant, even ten years ago. Rather the assumptions of the essay were what Nietzsche would term "unseasonable." Hiatt was appealing to a moral sensibility that largely did not and still does not exist in his readers. He appealed to what we all value in common, and he talked about a shared predicament. His essay addressed us not as individuals with diverse interests and values, but as a society of doctors and patients at least minimally bound together in some fundamental way. It is this sense of the commonweal, of a shared, public good, that was and is dormant within us.

This book, like all writing on the justice of our health care system, is liable to a fate similar to Hiatt's essay. Justice is a difficult concept for most Americans, but not because we are uninterested in it. Rather the difficulty is because questions of justice speak to us as members of a collective and appeal to our moral likenesses, our commonness, our basic sense of ourselves as creatures with shared vulnerabilities and shared needs. To the extent that we can reawaken and sharpen this sense, arguments about justice in health care can be engaged. To the extent that it remains

1

dormant, all arguments about a just health care system will be perceived as simple extensions of an individualistic ethics and judged by criteria of individual rights, rules, and virtues. It is for this reason that arguments about a just health care system, posed in an age of individualism, must not only argue in the usual way for one or another principle of allocation. We must find a way, in addition, to show how the arguments are intended to work, and why they are appealing.

Thus the purpose of this book is twofold. The first (and obvious) purpose is an argument for certain principles of justice in health care allocation. Here the typical format of argument, objection, and counterargument is followed. The second (and less obvious) purpose of the book is to show, by exposition and example, the different senses of self and society implicit in the various notions of justice which are examined. This second task is essential, for no ethical argument can succeed without reference to the sort of moral beings we think we are, including perceptions of how we are related to others. All arguments for a more just health care system must be grounded in a true sense of these human relationships. Thus the title, *Rationing Health Care in America: Perceptions and Principles of Justice*, indicates attention to both the principles of justice which should guide our choices and the ideas of self and society which form the background for our thinking.

Philosophical medical ethics over the last decade has largely neglected the macro issues of justice in favor of the micro, individual dilemmas of life and death in intensive care settings. More importantly, philosophical ethical anallysis has assumed that the basic task of ethics is finding common principles to adjudicate moral differences. Such a view of the task is satisfactory, so far as it goes, but it neglects the perceptions of self and society to which principles appeal. This book seeks to remedy that shortcoming. It sees the task of ethics in health care as the articulation of principles which will be true to our most basic moral perceptions. Probing these background perceptions will give us a better sense of both the strengths and the limitations of the principles we use.

The arguments presented here are, I believe, solid, but they are neither definitive nor exhaustive. The problems of health care allocation span several fields, including clinical medicine, health policy and economics, political philosophy, and medical sociology, to say nothing of ethics. Philosophers, especially, may find the arguments incomplete, for I have not attempted to sniff out all of my assumptions or to anticipate every objection which might be made to my thesis. A full philosophical accounting of these issues would require several volumes, and I leave that to others with more skill and patience. The primary audience I wish to address is medical students, house officers, and physicians in practice, hospital administrators and others who make policy, and the variety of professional and preprofessional students who will be rationing health care over the next several decades.

Since one of the major barriers to an ethics of justice in health care is lack of good descriptions of our own health conditions and the choices we have, I have larded the text with a variety of health data, case studies, parables, and other scenarios of moral choice. Perhaps even the reader who accepts none of my conclusions will be able to push the inquiry further and more effectively after confronting this material.

Chapter 1, "The Reality and Necessity of Rationing," presents the background for the arguments which follow. Rationing is not a future possibility but a present reality. Reasons are given why allocation problems are likely to become more acute in the future.

Chapter 2 describes the predominance of ethical individualism, a morality which marks both personal health behaviors and physician conduct in America. The parable of the Good Samaritan is explored as a model of medical ethics and for its uses and limitations in moving toward a social ethics.

Chapter 3 is an examination of the way contemporary theories of justice rely on ethical individualism. John Rawls and Robert Nozick are discussed as examples of political philosophers who work with impoverished perceptions of moral selfhood. Adam Smith's notion of sympathy is offered as an instance of a more realistic view, to which principles of justice can appeal.

Chapter 4 articulates principles of justice which are more true to the social sense of self. A variety of objections to the right to health care are considered. A carefully defined and socially grounded right to health care emerges as the measure of justice. The affirmation of principles of justice converts the bare fact of our social relatedness into an intentional social union—a community. The principle of need-based equity is discussed as a bridge between identified and statistical lives.

Chapter 5 presents an outline for a system of rationing health care. Conflicts within the role of the physician are explored. An equitable and accessible system of preventive services and primary care is endorsed. It is argued that efficacy and utility should be guiding criteria for secondary and tertiary services.

Finally, the case studies discuss rationing in three contexts: life-threatening situations, ambulatory care, and in the larger sphere of competing health care programs.

1. The Reality and Necessity of Rationing

American health care is full of contradictions. We spent $250,000 to keep Barney Clark alive, tethered to an air pump, for 112 days of "encumbered twilight" in Salt Lake City.[1] Meanwhile, in cities like Detroit, Boston, and Raleigh the infant mortality rate, frequently related to basic nutritional and perinatal care, has begun to rise. So far the federal government has contributed over $240 million to develop the artificial heart,[2] while at the same time cutting the programs which provide for the needs of indigent mothers and infants.

With the advent of cyclosporins, many large medical centers are now preparing their facilities to offer heart, liver, and other organ transplant services, at a cost of hundreds of thousands of dollars per procedure. Simultaneously, large public hospitals in some Southern states are closing their emergency rooms on weekends in order to stem the flow of poor patients who use emergency rooms for primary care.[3]

Infertile couples can increasingly have their desire for children treated by in vitro fertilization and implantation techniques, at roughly $4,000 per attempt. Persons in chronic vegetative states sometimes have their kidneys and bowels washed, their lungs cleared, and their infections treated at public expense. While some seem to live needlessly, others seem to die needlessly. Eugene Barnes, a 32-year-old, unemployed, stab-wound victim, died in a San

5

Francisco hospital in February, 1985. He was turned away
from four other hospitals because he lacked health
insurance.[4]

These examples are but a fraction of the startling contrasts in health care in this country. The question which
finally must be answered is: Are these allocations of health
care just? But before proceeding to this question it is important to trace some of the history of how we came to be
where we currently are. Just or not, scenes like these are
bound to increase as pressures of cost containment and
efficiency make it even more evident who receives care and
who does not.

Escalating Costs

In the United States the cost of health care has been
rising at twice the rate of inflation over the past decade. In
1986 Americans are estimated to have spent $450 billion
for health care—more than $1,800 for every man, woman,
and child. Health care costs constituted almost 11 percent
of the Gross National Product for 1986, and health care is
now the nation's second largest industry.[5]

No single factor accounts for this steady rise in the cost
of health care. Medical, technological, professional, cultural, and other factors have all played a role. The items
discussed here are not exhaustive but they are some of the
most prevalent, and they indicate why allocation pressures
promise to increase for the foreseeable future.

The percentage of persons over 65 has risen steadily in
all industrialized countries during the past century. The
life expectancy at birth (1982) is now 71 for all males and
78 for all females in the U.S. By 1990 13 percent of the
population will be 65 or over, by 2040 it will rise to 23
percent.[6]

As the population ages, chronic disease becomes more
prevalent. Chronic diseases (rather than acute) are now the

most frequent cause of death in industrial societies. Heart attack, stroke, and cancer have replaced infectious diseases as the major causes of mortality. Setting aside the age factor, it is estimated that 50 percent of the civilian population of the U.S., excluding those in institutions, have one or more chronic conditions. It is also estimated that currently 80 percent of all health care resources in the U.S. are devoted to chronic disease, and this is likely to increase.[7]

As the population ages and chronic illnesses increase, disability increases as well. Thirty million Americans (14 percent of population) were reported to have dysfunction in 1978. Three quarters of these disabilities were major enough to affect the person's ability to work, manage a household, or attend school.[8]

Technology has also had a profound impact on health care costs. In the 1950s and 1960s, federal legislation promoted the use of technology-intensive, hospital-based services (Hill-Burton, Medicare, and Medicaid). Also, because it was assumed that physicians would not take the initiative in exploiting new medical technologies, Regional Medical Programs were launched to acquaint them with the latest procedures. In recent years, with rising health care costs, planners have sought ways to curtail the increase in hospital beds, services, and technologies. The hospital is now viewed as a powerful, nearly uncontrollable consumer of scarce resources.

It is uncertain how much of the increased cost of medical services is attributable to technology, but it is a significant portion. For example, hospital expenditures rose from $3.9 billion in 1950 to $135.5 billion in 1982. Thirty percent of this increased hospital cost is directly attributable to new science and technology.[9]

Technology has, of course, affected the very character of disease, permitting greater control, yet not always being curative. The dramatic breakthroughs with infectious diseases have been cheap and relatively simple to administer. Lewis Thomas has given the name "halfway technologies" to those which are especially expensive, but not curative or only partially effective, such as renal dialysis.[10] Partial technologies have permitted the survival of more or less serverely disabled persons who previously would have died. Other invasive and expensive technologies have proved to be inefficacious—gastric freezing for peptic ulcer or adrenal-ectomy for essential hypertension.

In brief, one way to express the problem of allocation of health care is to say that there are scarce resources in relation to human needs. And this scarcity is exacerbated by the escalating costs of care and the greater demands for care by an increasingly aged, chronically ill, and disabled society which is attracted to the uses of high technology.

But the situation is further complicated by three additional forces: financing schemes that work on fee for service and cost reimbursement bases; traditions of professional ethics that encourage treatment even for very marginal benefits; and American health utopianism.

Fee for service medicine rewards the physician with more money for more services and, especially, for more procedures. Thus there is a financial incentive to the physician for doing more rather than less. Cost reimbursement financing rewards physicians and hospitals with more revenue for generating higher costs. Finally, physicians, hospitals, and many patients are protected from direct concern about cost by third parties who actually pay the bills, mainly Medicare, Medicaid, Blue Cross-Blue Shield, and commercial insurance companies.[11] While Health Maintenance Organizations, and the new Diagnosis Related Groups' prospective payment scheme of Medicare, are changing these traditional financing patterns, many suggest that they may create even greater disparities in access to health care as hospitals are forced to economize and accept fewer uninsured patients.

While economists tend to place great weight on financing schemes, ethical traditions within medicine also contribute to rising costs. A maximalist philosophy has dominated

American medicine since the end of the Second World War. Under this philosophy, it is considered anathema to do less than everything possible to forestall death. Frequently discussed as a sanctity of life ethic, the practices of maximal effort to sustain life easily slip into a vitalistic "life at all costs" position.[12] In a less dramatic vein, Aaron Wildavsky calls this the "Medical Uncertainty Principle." To satisfy physician insecurity and patient anxiety, "there is always one more thing that might be done—another consultation, a new drug, a different treatment."[13] Those who have advocated or practiced restraint and more reasonable uses of resources have not infrequently had their motives or professional competence questioned. We are a society which is uneasy about death and, substituting longevity in this life for spiritual reassurance of the next, have imbued the priesthood of medicine with a maximalist ethic of preservation.

Clearly a part of the maximalist ethic is not attributable to doctors' authentic convictions but to so-called "defensive medicine," that is, to physicians doing much more than is necessary in order to defend themselves from dissatisfied patients and consequent malpractice suits. Another factor contributing to a maximalist ethic is high public expectations about medicine's ability to improve and enhance life generally. Problems formerly within the purview of priests, parents, friends, or the courts have been shifted to the province of the doctor. The resulting medicalization of much of personal and social life has been well described by Ivan Illich, in his learned rant against organized medicine, *Medical Nemesis.*

> In a medicalized society the influence of physicians extends not only to the purse and the medicine chest but also to the categories to which people are assigned. Medical bureaucrats subdivide people into those who may drive a car, those who must stay away from work, those who must be locked up, those who may become

soldiers, those who may cross borders, cook, or practice prostitution, those who may not run for the Vice-Presidency of the United States, those who are dead, those who are competent to commit a crime, and those who are liable to commit one.[14]

Thus, while chronicity, disability, and technology are major factors in the rising cost of health care, economic, ethical, and cultural forces also play an important role. In part, what we face in health care costs are the burdens of our previous successes in preventing early death. Chronic diseases are more expensive to treat and people on average live to develop greater degrees of morbidity. Premature death, while tragic, is the great medical economizer. Meanwhile, a flexible concept of human nature and an inflated notion of health press our expectations beyond realistic limits.

Yet increasing costs in health care are only part of the problem, for even greater costs might be acceptable if everyone's health care needs were being met. And this is far from the case.

Limited Access

Not everyone benefits from the current health care system. The poor, non-white, elderly, together with those who live in urban ghettos or remote rural areas, are in the poorest health and receive the fewest benefits. Meanwhile, the elderly are spending out of pocket a larger percentage of their total income than before Medicare was enacted. At any one time, there are over 25 million uninsured Americans but as many as 34 million are uninsured for some period during the year; 18 million are without insurance for the entire year.[15] Among the under 65 population in the rural South, more than one-third have no hospitalization insurance, including Medicaid.[16] For black Americans the infant mortality rate is almost double that of whites.[17]

The problems of access are problems of both financial and geographic access. Some who live close to medical facilities cannot afford to pay or are uninsured. Some for whom money is not a barrier must travel long distances to find medical attention. Some are limited or denied care on both counts.

Many Americans assumed that with the passage of Medicaid in 1965 practically no one was without health care insurance. The actual situation is very different. Categorical restrictions and income eligibility cut-offs in most states, accelerated by the Reagan Medicaid cuts of 1981, mean that 60 percent of those who currently fall below the poverty level are not covered by Medicaid.[18] As one would expect, the uninsured use health services only about half as much as the insured, and receive about half as much hospital care, in spite of the fact that the uninsured perceive themselves as being in worse health than the insured.[19] This perception is accurate. Low-income families show a greater prevalence of many chronic diseases. For example, the poor have 65 percent more hypertension, 85 percent more instances of hearing impairments, and, in the 45–64 age group, twice as much heart disease.[20]

While geographic distribution of physicians has improved over the past two decades, there are still major shortages in many rural and inner-city areas. For example, in Mississippi, 105 of the state's 170 obstetricians live in just five of the state's eighty-two counties, while fifty-one counties have no obstetrician at all.[21] An estimated 20 million Americans live in areas classified as greatly underserved, that is, where there is less than one primary care physician for every 2,000 persons and more than 20 percent of the population is poor. Here, as expected, high rates of infant mortality, chronic conditions, and substandard health conditions prevail.[22] There are presently over 2,000 parts of the country designated as Health Manpower Shortage Areas.[23]

Unfortunately physician inaccessibility has another face as well. Physician participation in the federal programs to assist the underserved is limited. Roughly 32 percent of doctors in medical specialities, 15 percent of those in surgical specialties, and 40 percent of psychiatrists do not treat any Medicaid Patients.[24] Also, half of all Medicare claims are taken by physicians on condition that the patient promises to cover charges over and above the Medicare reimbursement rates.[25] So while many physicians participate in federal programs to increase access, a sizeable group do not, and those who do may require additional payment from patients. The reasons for physician non-participation vary, but at least in part they derive from traditions of medical individualism and professional sovereignty which will be discussed in the next chapter.

The composite picture is one of major inequities in access to care. This fact, in itself, however, is not a full statement of the problem. The problem of justice arises because lack of access to health care is a major factor in ill health. For some this will seem too obvious to merit discussion, for others a questionable and inflated assumption.[26] Yet the point is crucial to the argument, for if health care were a neutral or insignificant factor in a person's health status, no question of injustice could arise. One is not being wronged by being denied access to a service which is ineffective. Yet health care is a significant component in how healthy we are. This claim is, of course, much stronger with some sorts of services than others, for example, very strong for treatment of strep throat and less strong for physician counseling of remediation of poor health practices. On the whole, however, it is undeniably the case that access to health services makes a difference. The impact cannot be precisely measured but it is significant.

Between 1968 and 1980 in the U.S., deaths from influenza and pneumonia dropped by 53 percent, deaths from tuberculosis dropped by 52 percent, and deaths from diabetes by 31 percent.[27] Between 1970 and 1978 age-adjusted mortality rates in general dropped twice as fast as over the ten previous years.[28] Both these gains are attributable at least in part to the gains in health care access inaugurated in the mid-1960s by Medicare and Medicaid. Since Medicaid also made services available to many indigent mothers and their children, the overall infant death rate has declined from 24.7 per 1,000 live births in the mid-1960s to 12.5 per 1,000 live births in 1980.[29] Finally, the improved services offered by the Indian Health Service can be credited with at least a portion of the 70 percent reduction in the infant mortality rate among American Indians between 1960 and 1979.[30]

This is not to argue that all medical services are beneficial nor that we may not be using too many services in some areas of health care. Health, under any definition, depends upon both individual and social virtues. Health is a function of many variables—hygiene, stress, personal habits, living conditions, nutrition, exercise, as well as access to a physician, hospital, or other services. The studies do show, however, that basic health care does make a marked difference in many areas of life and that there are major disparities in the degree to which persons in our society can obtain it.

Access to health care is distributed inequitably, favoring the insured, the wealthy, and the white. In addition, the burdens of paying for health care are also distributed unevenly, but with the greatest burden borne by the less well served. Current federal tax laws exclude from taxable income employers' contributions to their employees health insurance. This amounts to a tax subsidy for those with employer-sponsored health insurance, the lost revenue for which totaled $29 billion in 1982.[31] Moreover, the benefits of this tax subsidy are distributed unevenly, with the greatest tax savings going to those with the highest incomes and the best health insurance policies. In sum, in 1982 the federal government spent $36 billion on health care for the poor,[32] while providing $29 billion in health-related tax subsidies for the middle and upper classes.

So the question of justice is raised, unambiguously and forcefully, by the statistics themselves. Is it just when some members of a society receive the best health care anywhere in the world while others receive little or nothing? To answer this question in more than a superficial way will require a more detailed digging into the ethical, cultural, and economic traditions which inform our political and medical systems. This is the task of subsequent chapters. For now we must focus on a more elementary fact, that we are in the United States currently rationing health care and have been for some time.

Rationing: A Current Practice

This is a hard fact to face. Some of the most astute observers of American health care shy away from it. Aaron and Schwartz, for example, after investigating allocation practices in British hospitals, conclude that if and when it comes to the U.S. "Rationing will inevitably be a painful prescription."[33] This implies that rationing is not now going on, which is false. It is not rationing by a central authority, but it is rationing nonetheless—rationing by price, and in secondary instances by disease (as in federal coverage for renal dialysis and Hanson's disease) or by age (as in Medicare) or by race (as in the Indian Health Service), and so on. But access is mostly contingent on having a way to pay for it, either out of one's own resources or with some form of insurance. The essential point is that allocation by price is a rationing scheme—one which we have easily accepted in health care as an extension of a basic economic philosophy, and one which largely absolves any particular persons from responsibility for the results. Since no one actually decided to exclude the poor (as it is their lack of money that excludes them, not our actions) no one is responsible and no one is to blame. It is the genius of laissez-faire health care that it orders the priorities of care by not ordering them, that is, by letting the market forces decide who gets what. This enables us to say, regarding the outcomes, that we are all innocent of ill will or prejudice against those who cannot compete. In the end, since no one is in charge, no person or sets of persons are really responsible. The standard line is that these inequities are unfortunate but not unfair. The fairness or unfairness of this system is to be judged as we proceed. The essential thesis to keep before us now is that we do ration, and that inevitably, we must ration health care by some means. The question is: Which means serve the ends of justice?

Yet even this thesis—that rationing is inevitable—needs argument. Five objections can be lodged against it.

Some argue that greater efficiency can eliminate the need for allocating health resources.[34] Proponents of this perspective like to point to "waste" in the system and believe that if the "fat" were trimmed all would be well. Duplication of diagnostic tests, unwarranted surgery, lack of effective physician policing, and excess hospital beds are favorite (and legitimate) examples cited by those who believe efficiency can eliminate the need to ration.

Yet several factors argue against proponents of efficiency. First, health care needs are not determined independently of those who meet those needs, namely physicians. Scarcity (as unmet needs) is to a large degree controlled not by objective tests but by complex physiological, psychological, and symbolic forces in the interaction between physicians and patients. Here efficiency is in the service of a slippery and largely subjective goal. This leads to a second objection, namely, that it is far from clear that health care needs can be satiated at all. While we may assent intellectually to functional notions of health and minimally adequate notions of health care, our health behavior is less rational. Health at one level seems to stimulate greater needs for more services at a higher level. Thus, many people, free from fear of early death from infectious diseases, flock to high-level wellness clinics, exercise programs, psychotherapy, stress reduction, or in extreme cases, cosmetic surgery. Definitions of health, and therefore of health needs, seem remarkably fluid and without clear limits. Finally, a good deal of health care cannot be rationalized (or made more efficient) because it serves to alleviate no identifiable malady at all, but satisfies a more fundamental human need for attention, concern, and a collaborative relationship with a figure of beneficent power. Efficiency will be of limited value until we can answer: "Efficiency in the service of what?" Until then efficiency will be merely a tool, and a tool at odds with some of the reasons persons seek health care from the outset.

A second objection to rationing is that technology will eventually bail us out of shortages.[35] Those who espouse this way of thinking draw from the rhetoric (but usually not the wisdom) of Lewis Thomas. Thomas is eloquent about the inexpensiveness of genuine technologies such as the polio vaccine, which can truly eliminate an illness. He points out that the most expensive medical technologies, such as renal dialysis, are usually only partially effective. Thomas is, of course, right about the differences between total and partial technologies, but those who invoke his insight as a solution miss the major point. The root problem of allocation is not a technical problem at all. The issue of how to maintain or restore health more effectively is only secondary. The more urgent issue has to do with how to define health, how to adjudicate needs, and whose needs will count. Once these issues are clarified, technologies—halfway or total—will be useful. The reliance on technology is, in the end, susceptible to the same sort of fallacy as reliance on efficiency. Both present an important means as if it were the end or goal sought. Technology in the service of what? In the case of polio vaccines or CT scanners the answer seems clear. In the case of rhinoplasty, *in vitro* fertilization, artificial hearts, or psychotropic drugs the answer is more ambiguous.

Emphasis on technological wonders feeds our expectations for a health utopia and affects our willingness even to consider the degree to which we may be in part responsible for our own health problems. Garrett Hardin has given classic expression to this general phenomenon in relation to the population problem, but it applies equally well to the medical realm. Rationing is a "no technical solution" problem,[36] a problem of the human condition which depends to a minor degree on our ingenuity and technical intelligence and to a major degree on our moral grasp of our situation.

The third objection against rationing health care is that 11 percent of the GNP is not too much. When health care is weighed against other, more dubious, uses of our resources it seems well worth the expense. Proponents challenge us to say why 11 percent of the GNP is excessive. Here the argument is that rationing in health care is artifically created by treating other expenditures acritically, or as sacrosanct. If health care were to get its fair share, rationing in health care could be avoided. A nephrologist has put the point forcefully in relation to the patients he sees.

> How expensive is dialysis in relation to other things that government—and hence, society—undertakes? For example: public schools, aircraft carriers, super highways, military defense in outer space, education for physicians, bureaucracy, national parks, military aid to dictatorships, and so on and on. I believe we can afford it.[37]

There is an important point here. Just how much is too much is a social and political issue appropriately decided by political processes in which the worth of competing programs can be measured. We should not arbitrarily say 11 percent or 15 percent or even more is too much without a careful balancing of health care with other social priorities. Yet the pressure to cut costs is not coming from a single sector of our society. Few would disagree that— worthy as some cases may be—considered as a whole, current costs are out of proportion to value. We are buying, in many

cases, health care at the margins, paying more and more
for less and less. International comparisons add weight to
this view. Brian Abel-Smith argues that we in the U.S. are
the "odd man out" among industrialized nations for our
inability to control costs and with regard to the cost effectiveness of the services we buy.[38]

A fourth objection to the inevitability of rationing is
that capitalistic medicine will "outproduce" needs, creating
an excess that will filter down to everyone in society. Adam
Smith believed that only capitalism could vanquish scarcity and, through the "invisible hand," progress could
reconcile social inequity with adequate provision for the
poor.[39] This may be true, so long as the comparison for
adequacy one has in mind, as Smith did, is the starving
savage who must daily trust his skill and luck just to eat.
Any meager subsistence provided by industrial production
is probably more adequate than this.

In the recent past the operative assumption has been the
trickle down theory—i.e., Adam Smith applied to health
care—which assumes that redistribution could be affected
and scarcity eliminated by greatly increasing the aggregate
supply of physicians. Market pressures would then force
physicians to move into shortage areas. This would at least
ease problems of geographic access. Over the past decade
the total physician supply has increased enormously and
there is some feeling that a surplus exists. Yet great problems of geographic access still remain.

The reason for this is that the American health care
system, even with the recent pro-competition emphasis,
does not obey classic supply-and-demand economics. While
some still like to invoke the free enterprise ethos, health
care is carefully subsidized and protected in this country
by a variety of powerful social and professional forces. The
suppliers (doctors) can largely create their own demand for
services.

Finally, there are those who believe that rationing is
inherently evil and refuse to discuss it altogether. The well-

insured and the wealthy have not personally felt the effects of our current rationing scheme, which keeps it remote from their experience and safely associated with the British or other socialist or welfare health systems. For most of us who enjoy very good, and frequently more-than-necessary care, we fail to discern that our good fortune is bought, literally, at the price of maintaining a tacit system of allocation in which money (or its equivalent, insurance) guarantees access while lack of it guarantees sporadic, inferior, or no care. Bringing this forcefully to our attention is probably the most powerful argument that some form of health care allocation is necessary in all societies. The urgent question is which form.

Perhaps Aaron and Schwartz can be rewritten to reflect our situation: rationing will inevitably be painful, when we realize we are engaged in it and is already painful for those whose rationed share is inadequate. There are, however, powerful ethical and cultural forces which keep that realization at bay.

2. Ethical Individualism:
"The solitude of his own heart"

The difficulties we have in rationing health care in the United States are not merely difficulties of knowing how best to allocate our resources. They are difficulties that arise from our reticence and disability to *think* about rationing health care at all. The idea is foreign and slightly repugnant—foreign because we do not have a robust tradition of social ethics in America and repugnant because part of the individual ethics we live by has a very high place for both abundance and self-sufficiency. A vibrant social ethics is in some sense a response to scarcity and mutual vulnerability among citizens. So there should be little surprise that efforts to mount a consideration of distributive justice in health care should meet with resistance, both at the conceptual and emotional level.

Traditions of social ethics are not entirely absent in America. There are rich religious notions of community membership and political traditions of republican citizenship that can serve us well. These paradigms of social morality are, however, subservient and largely dormant in most discussions of justice. The social ethics which are discussed in essays and articles on rationing health care are usually simple extensions of individual morality. But the problem is not merely that justice is conceived as an extension of individual morality, but that this morality is highly *individualistic.* Under current views, the key concepts and images of justice are borrowed from a view of the person as independent and solitary and only tangentially related to others. In short, the current views are built upon an atomistic anthropology, a moral heritage in which answers to the question "What is good?" and "What is right?" are lodged definitively in a powerful image of the individual as the only meaningful level of moral analysis.

There is no better expression of this image of the individual than Philip Slater's parable in the "Preface" to his *The Pursuit of Loneliness: American Culture at the Breaking Point.*

Once upon a time there was a man who sought escape from the prattle of his neighbors and went to live alone in a hut he had found in the forest. At first he was content, but a bitter winter led him to cut down the trees around his hut for firewood. The next summer he was hot and uncomfortable because his hut had no shade, and he complained bitterly of the harshness of the elements.

He made a little garden and kept some chickens, but rabbits were attracted by the food in the garden and ate much of it. The man went into the forest and trapped a fox, which he tamed and taught to catch rabbits. But the fox ate up the man's chickens as well. The man shot the fox and cursed the perfidy of the creatures of the wild.

The man always threw his refuse on the floor of his hut and soon it swarmed with vermin. He then built an ingenious system of hooks and pulleys so that everything in the hut could be suspended from the ceiling. But the strain was too much for the flimsy hut and it soon collapsed. The man grumbled about the inferior construction of the hut and built himself a new one.

One day he boasted to a relative in his old village about the peaceful beauty and plentiful game surrounding his forest home. The relative was impressed and reported back to his neighbors, who began to use the area for picnics and hunting excursions. The man was upset by this and cursed the intrusiveness of human beings. He began posting signs, setting traps, and shooting at those who came near his dwelling. In revenge groups of boys would come at night from time to time to frighten him and steal things. The man took to sleeping every night in a chair by the window with a loaded shotgun across his knees. One night he turned in his sleep and shot off his foot. The villagers were saddened by this misfortune and thereafter stayed away from his part of the forest. The man became lonely and cursed the unfriendliness of his former neighbors. And all these troubles the man saw as coming from outside himself, for which reason, and because of his technical skills, the villagers called him the American.[1]

Unpacking some of the images in the parable of Slater's American will give us a working sketch of ethical individualism.

First, he prizes his independence and his privacy. Like another American, Henry David Thoreau, he wants to escape the "prattle" of his neighbors and seeks a solitary existence. Life in the wild is free of the constraints engendered by living in proximity to others. Freedom here is largely negative, not being interfered with by intrusive others. This coincides with the notion of rights which guides contemporary culture. Rights are thought to reside primarily within individual persons and are largely guarantees of personal liberty against outside coercion. That is, rights are largely negative, freedoms interpreted as lack of constraint from others. The primary image of others is as beings who constrict liberties, impose limits, create barriers, or otherwise inhibit authentic expressions of selfhood. The American, alone in the wild, is presumably freed from these moral evils to achieve some sort of self-actualization.

And the American is assisted in his quest by great ingenuity, which is the second striking feature of the hero of the parable. A modern Adam, the American not only constructs his own hut and invents an ingenious hooks-and-pulleys system; he tames wild creatures as well.[2] Ingenuity goes hand-in-glove with the virtue of self-sufficiency. Doing everything for oneself, this lack of dependence, comes into play so that one need not be morally indebted to the neighbor. And where no debts are owed, one can be free to relate to the neighbor on one's own terms. The American is again free, but this time free of the constraints of indebtedness or gratitude which previous kind acts incur.

This lack of moral indebtedness, bought from total self-reliance, means that all acts of relating to others may be seen as acts of charity or philanthropy. If one is sovereign over the provision of his or her own needs, no debts are owed to anyone. All moral acts of relating to others can, therefore, be freely chosen or freely rejected. All relations with others are acts of supererogation. The American owes duties to no one but himself, and self-expression is seen then as the most authentic of personal codes. Independence, privacy, ingenuity, self-reliance, sovereignty over needs and wants, and lack of social obligations to others all fit neatly together here into a portrait of American individualism in the extreme.

Technology also plays a part. Machines are considered good or, at worst, morally neutral. Lacking Thoreau's mystical regard for nature, the American of the parable assumes that the despoiling of both the natural and personal environment can be rectified by technological novelty. The irony, of course, is that each new technology (axes, hooks and pulleys, tamed foxes, shotguns) in turn creates even greater problems—some of them insoluble and the damage from them irreversible. The theme is not the evil of technology, but that technology without moral wisdom is destructive of the human good it should serve. Reliance on technology also makes the American susceptible to an excessive optimism about his abilities and precludes the recognition of some core insights of morality, such as failure, finitude, and tragedy.

The key theme of the parable is the American's lack of

self-knowledge. He has no insight into himself or his predicament. This lack of insight relates directly to his solitariness. Other people are mirrors for our self-knowledge, and the man in the parable has no others. Logically and experientially, one's person is distinctive and identifiable, and one's values discernible because of the history and traditions which emerge from relationships with others. This simple fact—that we are who we are and come to know who we are only by virtue of relating to others—is the crucial missing element for the character of the parable. He often acts in ignorance of the way his actions thwart his own aims, and this is because he has lost the neighborly prattle. There are, of course, good neighbors and bad, but even the most reclusive of hermits usually has a divine prattle to count on to orient the self. It is the American's attempt at a sheer, radical independence that is so shattering to moral self-awareness.

Ironically, in the end the American who sought to be the active agent in all his activities saw no agency except what lay outside himself. He has no other sense of how others act on him than as their victim. The enormous degree of self-involvement in his misfortunes bypasses him altogether, and all problems are perceived as caused by others infringing on his freedoms.

The parable can also be read as a search for privacy. Privacy is a feature of life in community, a dimension which presupposes relationships as an abiding context. The fallacy of the American, in this vein, is that he seeks privacy in isolation from community and what he finds is loneliness.

Yet even the American of this parable, caricature as he is of our sensibility, is not without a veiled expression of his need for community. He does curse the "unfriendliness" and indifference of his former neighbors, signaling a vulnerability for companionship and fellow-feeling. It is important that the American expresses this out of his own need and not as a choice to be gracious or friendly, which would turn fellowship into largesse. Even so, it is not the expression of need but the recognition of it in oneself and others that is of moral importance, and it is precisely this recognition that is absent.

This thorough-going independence, distrust of society, and aversion to social relationships as confining and inauthentic was definitively expressed by Ralph Waldo Emerson in his essay "Self-Reliance." "Society everywhere is in conspiracy against the manhood of every one of its members," he said, adding that society is nothing but a "joint-stock company in which the members agree, for the better security of his bread to each shareholder, to surrender the liberty and culture of the eater."[3] Slater's American is the direct descendant of Emerson and Thoreau, but stripped of the moderating influences of the transcendentalist philosophy which valued and cultivated self-awareness.

Self-Reliance for Health

The parable of the American is a narrative that can be applied in part to both patient and physician behaviors. Our infatuation with and reliance on medical technology is the most obvious parallel, but it is also probably the least important. More central are our individualistic attitudes about health, illness, and responsibility for health care.

Leon Kass, John Knowles, and Ivan Illich, though strange bedfellows in other ways, are similar in their insistence that health lies within the province of individual responsibility.[4] Their common thesis, variously formulated, is on one level a proper corrective to the opposite assumption, namely that health can be guaranteed as a social and political right through ever-increasing medical progress. Yet each of these authors, in his own way, throws us back on ourselves as a solitary entity and invokes self-reliant behavior as the key to success in problems of ill health. Illich is unquestionably the most stridently individualistic of the three, and he comes closest to endorsing something like an unvarnished version of Slater's American. While Knowles and (especially) Kass are more balanced commentators on our moral sensibility, they are included here because they seem to see no alternative to reliance on doctors and medical progress other than an evocation of old-fashioned self-reliance. Missing is any sense that in the alternating rhythms of assigning responsibilities, essential aspects of the problem get lost. All three of these commentators are so concerned to reform and curtail the notion of health that they neglect to remark on the dynamics of total dependence/total independence that seem to mark our attitudes about health like extreme pendular swings of our moral sensibility.

Like the American in the parable, we often assume that in health and health care, either someone else is totally responsible for us or we are totally responsible for ourselves. Indeed, our attitudes seem to fluctuate between a radical sovereignty over our behavior when we are healthy and a radical dependence or passivity when we are sick. Thus we argue vehemently for the right to smoke, drink excessively, overeat, and engage in other damaging behaviors without social interference, but then assume unquestioningly the blameless and passive "sick role" when we are ill. This is precisely parallel to Slater's American, who sees no agency except that which was outside himself, and whose role as victim is the correlate of his assumptions of total freedom and independence.

This health behavior dovetails beautifully with the germ theory of disease causation. Germs invade, from the outside, attacking innocent and unsuspecting victims. Social, or even individual causal factors are ignored, so that the impurity can be isolated as to cause, encapsulated as to locus, and finally eradicated.

So with regard to Kass, who is the most eloquent of the champions of individual responsibility, we should accept gratefully his important corrective to an overblown and utopian ideal of health. But we must not seek a simple solution in the overtones of a self-reliance ethics which lards his essays. We need not choose between these alternatives. If self-reliance for health can be seen to be grounded in a more fulsome social sense of self, perhaps we can return to this and other virtues with fresh appreciation. As it stands, we are too enamored of self-reliance as a romantic ideal to place Kass's corrective in a proper context.

So the problem here is not that our attitudes about health are precisely those of the American of the parable. They are not, and often they are radically different. But all too frequently Americans are prone to espouse a health utopianism that evokes an acritical individualism as a counterpoint. We need not choose between the World Health Organization definition of health as complete psychosocial and physical well-being provided to us by others, and a minimalist, physiological definition of health as species well-functioning, for which each of us individually is totally responsible.[5] Unfortunately, a good deal of the literature revolves around this mutually reinforcing set of ideals. Between these two options there is little to choose from. For while one bespeaks an impractical ideal for health, the other tends to reduce health to a sheer minimalism. But more importantly, neither can support an adequate view of self to ground a theory of distributive justice. Both distort the nature of our relationships with others, weighing them too heavily or too lightly. The extent of our devotion to ethical individualism, like that of Slater's American, is profound, and profoundly influences our perceptions of health and proper health behaviors.

Individualism in Medical Ethical Codes

Physician attitudes and behaviors are also illuminated by Slater's parable. The history of American medical codes of ethics, for example, clearly shows the characteristics of individualist thinking, not only with what they say, but also with what they imply. It is one thing to examine codes for their explicit moral content, their principles and rules, and their advice to practitioners. It is quite another thing to look at codes for what they suggest about who the doctor is, who patients are, and what is thought to be the proper role of each. Sometimes exclusions are as important as inclusions in codes, and assumptions made by the authors of codes are equal in significance to written expressions. Both sorts of analysis are important.

The "Code" of the American Medical Association of 1847 is a good place to begin.[6] It was the first non-European formulation, and it also marks the beginning of the long ascendency of allopathic medicine over homeopathy, Thomsonianism, and a variety of other practices which persisted through the nineteenth century and, in some instances, well into the twentieth. As such it is a benchmark of professionalism for American medicine.

There are many notable things about this "Code": unlike current moral formulae in medicine, it speaks to character and does not merely list principles; it lists not only duties of physicians to patients but includes a complementary list of duties patients owe to doctors; and it contains an eloquent section on the duties of physicians to the general public. As contrasted with many twentieth-century lists of principles, the 1847 "Code" is a generous statement about the moral goals and motivations of a practitioner. Too frequently criticized as being merely etiquette, the "Code" evokes high ideals and appeals to noble character rather than simply urging intellectual assent to legalistic rules.

The signal aspect of this "Code," however, is that it assumes that the moral standards which should apply to physicians are essentially a creation of the profession itself. That is, the assumption seems to be that the norms, proper though they may be, are not discovered, but invented by doctors. Doctors then invent their own rules of conduct which can be changed as they see fit. The picture here is one of sovereignty over one's obligations to others, not as in the parable because others interfere, but because the nature of professional morality is such that one can exercise hegemony over what even counts as an obligation or duty. The opening paragraph of the "Code" states that a physician's obligations to the sick are all the more weighty "because there is no tribunal other than his own conscience, to adjudge penalties for carelessness or neglect."[7] This is a striking and far-reaching claim as it arrogates to a pinnacle of power individual conscience and claims an exclusiveness of judgment. It does not make an empirical claim that only a physician, by virtue of expertise of knowledge, will be able to judge carelessness or neglect. Rather the claim here is a metaethical one, an assertion about the nature of morality and the person who seeks to be moral. Morality is finally to rest with individual conscience; that is the bedrock of professional ethics for doctors, as this "Code" would have it.

There are, to be sure, lists of duties which physicians owe both to individual patients and to the public, but it must be remembered that these duties did not originate in some common bond between physicians and others. They are rather self-assumed duties which physicians impose upon themselves and over which each physician alone adjudges himself or herself to be in or out of accord. The role which others (patients and the public) have here is merely as the recipient of duties, not as in any way enjoying a previous human bond which grounds the physician's particular duties and in no way influencing either the content or the canons of excellence. On examination, the "Code" of 1847 has a remarkable affinity to the individualism of Slater's American, not so much in explicit content but in the presumptions from which the duties derive. It is finally the sovereign self which is the origin and judge of professional behavior here.

The AMA Code of 1847 underwent minor revisions in 1903, 1912, and 1947, but it was not until 1957 that a major change was made. The 1957 statement is not a code at all in the technical sense but several "Principles of

Medical Ethics."[8] The elegance of the older formulation is here replaced with terse statements, not actually of principles but more often of rules of prudential conduct. It retains most of the assumptions of professional sovereignty but deletes the nobility and appeals to character which gave the 1847 "Code" a touch of high-mindedness and respect. Moreover, the 1957 statement adds an assertion of prerogative absent from the earlier "Code." Section 5 of the 1957 "Principles" states that "A physician may choose whom he will serve."[9] This is clearly recognizable as fully in keeping with the tradition of self-imposed obligations described earlier and consistent with a moral life insulated from significant relations with others, both in its origins and its meaning. If one may truly choose whom one will serve, then every helping act may be interpreted as an act of charity, of supererogation. If there are no *a priori* duties to anyone except those freely chosen by the professional, then the sum of morality is largesse—there are no obligations except those one *chooses* to acknowledge. Loyalty, obligation, and duty lose all their usual force and become extensions of the will and results of the free choice to serve.

The point here is that this statement of "Principles," like the 1847 "Code," appeals to the physician as a sovereign and solitary agent, master of his own moral sensibility and in willful control over to whom and to what extent he is obligated. The "Principles" achieve a remarkably close affinity with the American of the parable, who sought to make every relationship with others a chosen one and its obligations and binding commitments calculated in advance and curtailed according to a deliberate measure.

Occasionally the AMA standards have been interpreted and applied to contemporary ethical problems, usually in the form of Opinions and Reports of the Judicial Council. The 1971 *Opinions and Reports* dealt with the issue of truth-telling, or disclosure of information under the heading "Prognosis":

The physician should neither exaggerate nor minimize the gravity of a patient's condition. He should assure himself that the patient, his relatives or his responsible friends have such knowledge of the patient's condition as will serve the best interests of the patient and family.[10]

This maxim reflects a traditional ethics based on the assumptions of private prerogatives. It is, to be sure, commendable to have the best interests of the patient and the family in clear and prominent focus. But the axial issue is whose notion of "best" is the appropriate one? And on what value assumption does that notion rest? According to this *Opinion* the physician presumes to make this decision as a matter of professional competence. Thus, relating a diagnosis—or whether to disclose it at all—is thought to be a privilege entirely within the professional's individual discretion.

It is not simply that physicians are thought to know more than others regarding the diagnosis, or that they should know best how to communicate what they know; in the individualist moral tradition, that knowledge is presumed to warrant a moral corollary, *viz.*, that professional knowledge of diagnosis is also knowledge of what is *good for* the patient. And what is good for the patient is thought to need no other court of adjudication than what the physician in his moral self-sufficiency decides.

The point is not that this statement from the Judicial Council is somehow wrong. Rather it is that the grounds for deciding right and wrong have been eliminated from public or community view and placed within an isolated conscience.

The 1980 AMA "Principles of Medical Ethics" are the most recent formulation of American medical morality.[11] Generally, this document perpetuates the tradition described above. It expresses prerogatives for self-regulation, while stressing the autonomy of the individual practitioner. Patient welfare is said to be the aim and purpose of the "Principles," but only a vague sense of what this welfare might mean or how a physician might protect it is indicated. Moreover, there are a number of conspicuous omissions from the document, not the least of which is no mention of social justice in the distribution of physician services and no affirmation of the equality of patients as persons. The overall impression of the 1980 "Principles" is thereby of a union or guild ethics, a statement made by craftsmen to protect their self-interest and in which their prerogatives and rights form the central motif. The listed duties and obligations are thought to be self-imposed and freely assumed. They do not appear in any way as acknowledged duties based on a previous relationship of responsibility between physicians and the general public. In fact, there is no lively sense of the common good at all, except as this might be a spinoff from individual good works. Rather than reflect a larger cultural tradition of ethics, the "Principles" are written as if they were the *creatio ex nihilo* of doctors. It is in this deep sense that codes of ethics within medicine have traditionally reflected an ethics fully autonomous and professionalized and an ethos of moral sentiments severely attenuated in both scope and depth. From such a tradition of ethics and its underlying ethos have come our conventional notions of doctor-patient relationships.

Images of Virtue: Individual Heroism

We have difficulty as Americans with resource allocation at two levels—in the first place in knowing how to ration, but more importantly in being able to think about rationing as a moral activity at all. The absence of any strong social ethics and the dominance of ethical individualism over public or social traditions make our deliberations difficult and "unseasonable."

Persons do not think and perceive morally through formal statements or a cognitive grasp alone. Intellectual assent to doctrines of morality are probably far less important to our ethics than the figures which animate the moral imagination—saints, heroes, exemplars, models, and archetypes of virtue who through their deeds, and their sayings about their deeds, capture moral integrity concretely and preserve it for us in parable, story, or metaphor. Practical disciplines like ethics must have embodiments of "the good," not just abstract norms. In this sense it is more important to know who someone's heroes are than what principle he or she espouses. Iris Murdoch says we can only choose in the world we can perceive,[12] and there is no aid to perception like the critical incident, or slice-of-life that *shows* as well as talks about goodness and virtue. While Kant may be convincing, Mother Teresa is moving, and we intuitively understand and remember what she is doing even if we do not entirely agree with her actions. It is through the remembrance and rehearsal of stories of virtue that most of us have our surest grounding for the norms to which we ascribe.[13] So it is to the moral imagination that I now turn to discuss the figures which enliven and give substance to our values.

The one figure of virtue which most forcefully and clearly has captured the imagination of physicians is the Good Samaritan. "Samaritanism" has, in fact, become shorthand in our culture to express those essential dimensions of physician morality which are the *sine qua non* of the profession. The parable of the Good Samaritan, as recorded in Luke 10:30–35, goes like this:

> A man was going down from Jerusalem to Jericho, and fell among robbers who stripped him and beat him, and departed leaving him half dead. Now by chance a priest was going down that road, and when he saw him he passed by on the other side. So likewise a Levite, when he came to the place and saw him passed by on the other side. But a Samaritan, as he journeyed, came where he was; and when he saw him he had compassion. And went to him and bound up his wounds, pouring on oil and wine, and set him on his own beast and brought

him to an inn, and took care of him. And the next day he took out two denarii and gave them to the innkeeper, saying, "Take care of him; and whatever more you spend, I will repay you when I come back."

There are many facets of this story but our interest here is centered on obvious ways in which the story is generally regarded as a moving one and a worthy paradigm for virtuous action. The Samaritan goes out of his way, at some cost to himself, to provide help for a perfect stranger who is in need. Yet instead of being treated as a parable, the story is frequently used as a moral norm. But problems arise when the-story-as-moral-norm is taken to exhaust the nature of moral obligation. As Judith Jarvis Thomson has pointed out, the heroic character of the Samaritan's action overshadows the sense of minimal decency which one should have been able to expect from the priest and the Levite.[14] And when that happens, the model for virtue is not "minimal decency," but "good Samaritanism" or even "supererogatory Samaritanism"—that is, an isolated individual act which is distinguished by heroic proportions of splendor and largesse.

The Good Samaritan ideal plays upon our sense of concern for the less fortunate but it does not, as usually interpreted, evoke our sense of interdependence and conviviality with the person who lies beaten on the road.

We are not told whether the robber's victim gave his consent to the Samaritan's assistance; and it may be important to consider why this detail might have been omitted, as we try to understand other details which were included.[15] Acts of supererogation within the tradition of Samaritanism need no consent; indeed, the very conditions which make an action supererogatory also make the conventional consent requirement trivial and out-of-place. That is why patients who come to physicians in the "sick role" may be perceived as in such distress that a formal consent, in turn, is thought to be superfluous or demeaning. If medicine is armed with the moral authority of "Good Samaritanism," there is no need to inquire about permission of appropriateness of treatment. Patients perceived as sick and vulnerable are not supposed to be capable of collaborative relationships. From the patient's point of view, because these acts of assistance and healing are gratuitous, it seems indecorous and graceless to question them. One does not ask a drowning man whether he wishes to be rescued; nor does a drowning man ask for the certified qualifications of his would-be rescuer. The metaphor of rescue, extended to large provinces of patient care, remains a major image which shapes physician ethics.

This is not to suggest that the story of the Good Samaritan is a faulty moral guide, but simply to point out that, when translated into the American imagination and placed within the ethos of medicine, the message of the story tends to look like philanthropy. What usually goes unnoticed in our appropriation of this story is that the Samaritan acts out of compassion. He does not act out of altruism or *noblesse oblige,* nor does he see his help as fulfillment of a duty, or an ideal, or even a free and noble act. We are told, rather, that he is *moved by compassion* upon seeing the man in the road. Compassion means literally "to feel with," and denotes a sense of identification and community. Compassion is not saccharine pity or demeaning self-righteousness to the less fortunate; neither is it associated with the charisma which forms part of the physician's traditional authority. Indeed, it is precisely these miscontruals which are offensive and insulting to the sick. Authentic compassion, on the other hand, engages one genuinely and empathetically in community with others.

To get a better sense of just how important the concept of compassion is, it may be helpful to consider how a utilitarian or a Kantian might rewrite the parable to express the essential aspect of morality as they see it.

The Good Samaritan, after weighing the consequences of helping this particular man versus others he might encounter (or selling his horse to give money to the starving in Africa), helped the beaten man on the road.

or

The Good Samaritan, not wanting to compound the harm done to an injured person by moving him, proceeded to Jericho and sent back a rescue party.

or

The Good Samaritan, realizing that the universal principle of beneficence is the most valid and cogent of moral maxims, helped the beaten man on the road.

Each of these versions, and many others which one could write under the sponsorship of a moral theory, obviously vitiates the force of the story, and probably would ensure its obscurity in the history of ethics.

So compassion is a key element of the story, and it is probably this unreflecting and uncalculated response that captures our attention and makes this a paradigm for medicine; indeed, the most powerful, sustaining image which medicine holds up to itself, even when misinterpreted as a norm rather than a parable.

Yet it is the lucid simplicity of the story that is also its limiting factor if we try to think about social justice and allocation. We must remember that the story of the Good Samaritan occurs in a context in which Jesus is teaching the meaning of the law, love your neighbor as yourself. The parable of the Good Samaritan is offered as an answer to the question of a lawyer, who seeks to justify his own actions, by asking, "Who is my neighbor?" And arresting and powerful as this story is as a guide to individual acts of rescue, it is not clear how we are to interpret its meaning for anything beyond one-to-one neighborliness. Indeed, the power of the story has become truly an arresting power, paralyzing our imagination to stretch beyond those whom we encounter as identified individuals in distress. Since doctors typically see patients one at a time, the parable has a direct translatability in the routines of clinical practice. So it is no wonder that social ethics has suffered, since the paradigm so easily focuses, and to some degree isolates, attention toward those individuals who are currently in view.[16]

To get a proper feel for just how confining this view is, we might again rewrite the parable to make it explicitly a problem of social justice. One version might go like this.

A man was going down from Jerusalem to Jericho, and fell among thieves, who stripped him and beat him, leaving him half dead. Likewise a priest and then a Levite, in turn, proceeded down the same road, and were also attacked and beaten. Then along came a Samaritan, and saw the three men beaten and left in the road. Knowing he could assist one, or at most only two, the Samaritan puzzled, "Who is my neighbor?"

We might speculate here about what difference it would make if the Samaritan were a surgeon or an internist, or about the severity of the wounds, or if the Levite had a Blue Cross card. But the basic point is that some of our most cherished metaphors of virtuous action will have to be altered if we are to see the issues as ones, not simply of benevolence, but also of justice.

As it stands, we have an individual ethics of robust proportions, but a dormant social ethics. Individual heroism seems to overshadow all other considerations. Rosalind Williams in a *New York Times* editorial entitled "Two Kinds of Ethics" pointed to the problem in the ironic actions of President Reagan, who "pays heartfelt tribute to Lenny Skutnik for risking his life to rescue a drowning woman who had lost her grip on a helicopter lifeline after a plane crashed into the Potomac River—in the midst of a speech espousing policies that would cut lifelines from people desperately trying to stay afloat amid economic disaster."[17]

Individualism and Moral Distance

Part of the problem of mounting any social ethics, and likewise the appeal of the parable of the Good Samaritan, is that we are moved by what we see and recognize, and by what is nearest to us in blood, age, status, and history. We are also moved by persons currently in distress far more than by the possible, even certain, distress of persons in the future. Thus crisis medicine has always outdistanced prevention for dollars and other resources.

Recently the father of a child in need of a liver transplant persuaded the American Academy of Pediatrics to let him plead for a liver at their professional meeting. The President of the United States did the same for another child on one of his regular Saturday radio broadcasts. Each of us with children would probably sacrifice a great deal, including our own lives, to save one of our own. Thomas Murray calls this the "rescue impulse,"[18] and it is clearly related to how close we are and how much we identify with, or can at least identify by name or face, those in distress.

Several years ago a volunteer rang my doorbell and asked for a signature on a petition and for a donation. His cause was hemophilia and he hoped to convince the state legislature to appropriate more funds for treatment. With a recent lecture on allocation of medical resources fresh on my mind I expressed doubts as to whether treatment of hemophilia —being very expensive, not curative, and benefiting only a handful of people—was the best way for the legislature to spend whatever portion could go to health care. My remarks were met by looks of dismay, then anger, and a long subsequent conversation revealed that this volunteer was no disinterested do-gooder, as anyone but an academic philosopher would have guessed from the start. His brother suffered from hemophilia. It was a humbling lesson in the power of identified lives over our helping instincts and the difficulties of entertaining a larger social perspective.

Hemodialysis for renal failure was for many years confined to acute care, until in 1959 Dr. Belding Scribner of the University of Washington perfected the arteriovenus shunt which allowed for a continuous access site for the general circulation. Scribner's shunt changed the nature of dialysis and made it reasonably effective for chronic as well as acute renal disability. By 1968 about 1,000 persons were receiving dialysis for chronic problems, but thousands of other persons were denied dialysis because the expensive dialysis machines were in short supply. The way universal coverage for dialysis was obtained for all patients with renal failure is another lesson in the power identified lives have over our moral sensibility.[19] In 1972 Congress passed Public Law 92-603, which amended Medicare to cover those under 65 suffering from end-state renal disease. The key action in persuading Congress was the dialysis of the Vice President of the National Association on Hemodialysis and Transplantation before the House Ways and Means Committee in November, 1971.[20] An identified life, with a face, a name, a history, and an office was an irresistible appeal.

Jonathan Glover gives a particularly chilling example of the moral impact of distance and proximity in recounting a scene from Nicholas Bethell's *The Last Secret*.[21] According to the Yalta Agreement, large numbers of Soviet citizens living in the West were forcibly deported to Russia. Herded onto trains by troops, many committed suicide, for those who arrived faced death or forced labor camps. The psychological and physical distance from the victims anesthetized the British Foreign Office official who defended this policy against numerous protests. However, when a single woman did manage to see this official, she clung to his knees crying and was spared.

On a more routine level, each of us can probably recount a tale of a racial or national prejudice being shattered by an encounter with a member of the maligned group, who could no longer be safely categorized at a distance, and

who we now felt to be like us in important ways. Distance
keeps our pet biases sealed from such testing and, as Glover
shows, sometimes makes victimization and suffering
possible.

Moral distance can be of many sorts. Stanley Milgram
has shown that visual and auditory contact with others will
lessen the degree of harm we are willing to inflict on them.[22]
Some writers have speculated on the impact a transparent
womb would have on our willingness to do abortions.[23] It
would almost certainly diminish our capacity to do them
easily. The temporal distance between our current lives
and the effects of the national debt or the disposal of
nuclear waste pushes these priorities to the background.
Moral distance can be created by technical or professional
language (as when an unborn human being is called a "con-
ceptus"), by dissimilarities in age or appearance (witness
our disregard for the elderly and racial minorities), and a
host of other factors.

Moral distance keeps us from looking at the inconsisten-
cies and contradictions in our health care system. While
President Reagan made his emotional appeal for a doomed,
single child and invoked a variety of flashy resources,
including an Air Force jet, he cut basic programs for poor
mothers and children whose names and plight he did not
know in any concrete way. While most parents would
sacrifice their lives for their own children, most are also
unwilling to forego a steak dinner or theatre tickets to feed
hundreds of starving children in Africa or press their Congressman for more funds to prevent early neonatal deaths
in Detroit. Why? Distance seems to blunt the moral imagination, and the lack of identified lives to whom to relate the
rescue impulse seems to paralyze social ethics altogether.
The impulse which seems to serve us so well in classic
Good Samaritan cases is confused or befuddled when three
persons lie beaten by the road and may be altogether
absent if we are confronted by the massive suffering of
hundreds or thousands with whom we cannot identify.

A probing essay into this phenomenon is the last chapter in Jonathan Glover's book *Causing Death and Saving Lives.* Glover speculates on what it would mean to be able to overcome the disabling aspects of moral distance in the guise of a "rationalist man."

Rationalist man would lack any of the distorting effects of the defense mechanisms [of moral distance]. He would respond emotionally to all the foreseeable reverberations across time and space of his acts and omissions just as much as to consequences immediately experienced.[24]

Glover is himself uncertain as to whether such a change in our ability to see all these things at a distance would be better, and he suggests, but does not argue, that some capacity for distancing ourselves from suffering may be a defense mechanism necessary for our psychic survival. Yet Glover would agree that the scope of our moral imagination at present is severely limited and can clearly be stretched beyond its almost reflexive concern with rescue medicine (and our most visible and vocal citizens) to those who suffer out of earshot and largely without names or faces.

Our interest in individual ethics is then, in part, attributable to the sorts of limits we have as human beings. We are temporal and spatial beings of finite resources, and suffering which is present to us will likely always give greater impetus to action than that which we do not experience directly. Yet the current American ethics of health care is, in addition, severely attenuated by long-standing and well-entrenched traditions of individualism. Alexis de Tocqueville perceived the danger of individualism in the American character almost 150 years ago. Tocqueville described the problem as rooted in a deep devotion to material well-being and economic measures of citizenship. Those who have acquired economic power "owe nothing to any man; they expect nothing from any man; they acquire the habit of always considering themselves as standing alone and they are apt to imagine that their whole destiny is in their own hands."[25] Tocqueville presents the hazards of our economic and political traditions as forgetfulness of one's history, a false sense of self-sufficiency, and solitude and alienation.

> Thus not only does commercial democracy make every man forget his ancestors, but it hides his descendants and separates his contemporaries from him; it throws him back forever on himself alone, and threatens in the end to confine him entirely within the solitude of his own heart.[26]

Working our way out of this confinement will no doubt require efforts to make invisible and distant persons more visible and present to us, but it will also require a more rigorous conceptual effort to attend to the social realities and social ethics we are prone to neglect.

3. Perceptions of Justice: Self and Society

Since rationing is a fact of life for health care in the U.S., we must ask if the current rationing scheme is morally justifiable. The problems of justice are not a natural or easy set of considerations. They are frequently smothered by our preoccupation with individual virtue and liberty. Social ethics, to the extent that it does find a place in our thinking, is derivative and secondary, almost an afterthought of a moral self which prizes independence, self-reliance and a negative freedom conceived as non-interference from others.

There is no more telling evidence for the correctness of this thesis than the images of self and society which emerge from contemporary political philosophers. For here we find that even the concepts of justice which are espoused by the two chief rival schools of thought are both deeply indebted to a view of the self which is atomistic and morally independent and a view of society as a derivative construction of solitary selves.

Rawls and the Social Contract Tradition

John Rawls is the most widely acclaimed among contemporary social contract theorists, and more than a few have attempted to derive a just system of health care from his writings.[1] Rawls' best known and most important work is *A Theory of Justice,* which aims to "present a conception of justice which generalizes and carries to a higher level of abstraction the familiar theory of the social contract as found, say, in Locke, Rousseau, and Kant."[2]

The question of justice arises, Rawls thinks, because we all know that we have interests that will conflict with the interests of others. Yet, it is beneficial to form and live in an organized society. Society should not only protect us in the pursuit of our interests against others who may interfere, it is also a positive avenue for furthering our own interests. Thus, in a plurality of interests and opinions about what is good or worthy of pursuit, rules and procedures must be enacted which will reconcile the need to live in society with the pluralistic nature of the interests of its citizens. Such rules will be the foundational principles of justice, the basis for the content of the social contract.

Rawls' concept of how we come to know such basic rules of justice is his contribution to the tradition of contract liberalism. Let us imagine, Rawls says, an "original position" in which individuals are under a "veil of ignorance," so that while they know they have interests, they do not know what those interests are. They only know that as people pursue different aims, their own needs and goals are likely to collide with others. Persons, under the veil of ignorance, are free, rational, and self-interested, but lack knowledge of any specific content of their interests. In such a position, Rawls asks, what would sensible people choose? His answer is two principles: (1) "each person is to have an equal right to the most extensive basic liberty compatible with a similar liberty for others"; and (2) "social and economic inequalities are to be arranged so that they are both (a) reasonably expected to be to everyone's advantage, and (b) attached to positions and offices open to all."[3] The principles are to be ranked in lexical order, so that (1) must be fulfilled before (2) and "liberty can be restricted only for the sake of liberty."[4] The reason these principles, and not others, are foundational is that they are principles which any rational, self-interested person would accept as the just basis of social exchange and interaction in the original position. It is also this characteristic which makes them, in Rawls' view, universal—any sensible, calculating individual would see them as ones he or she would affirm. Thus the consent of the citizens of society is achieved through the enactment of rules which rational, disinterested individuals would of necessity choose to maximize their freedom to pursue their own goals.

What interests us about Rawls and his justifiably renowned work is not the explicit principles he espouses or his justification of them. It is rather his starting point and the view of the self articulated there. Rawls' view of justice is grounded in the idea that human beings in their social role are primarily disinterested, calculating individuals. That is, in the beginning, at the crucial moments of choice, there are individuals who calculate about how best to form a social order. The assumption is that individuals precede, logically if not temporally (since the original position is hypothetical), any social belonging or sense of prior relatedness.

The difficulty with this is, in part, that the hypothetical character of the original contract tends to strip persons of the historical lineaments that give to contracts their locus, force, and binding power. The contract is presented as if it were at the beginning of things, *in illo tempore,* before history, and this renders the contract severely depleted of content. This is, of course, Rawls' aim, because universal assent to the contract is thought to necessitate an appeal to a formal characteristic of human beings, such as reason or self-interest, rather than an historical (and contingent) aspect, such as class, race, or endowments of intellect or wealth. But this logical strength is a practical weakness. Not only is the Rawlsian contract a hypothetical agreement that never happened, it is an agreement which could only be made by persons who never existed and never could exist. And this is a substantial weakness. The hypothetical nature of the contract removes it from history, but more importantly, the monodimensional contracting agents are not fulsome persons with whom we can identify, but logical constructs which we can merely apprehend as rational ideal types. We never were, nor will we ever be, stripped of the particularities of place, social role, and circumstance, because these are not mere accidental attachments to our essential (rational, self-interested) nature. These historical pecularities *are* us; they are the way we find our identity at all, and they require a social ambiance which is given rather than wholly chosen by acts of will.

What is in question here, then, is not whether Rawls' notion of justice is to be preferred over others. His notion is a congenial one. Rather, the issue is one of what kind of self it is that enters into society and makes the rules of justice. As is evident, the Rawlsian self is a thin, rational self, calculating its self-interest in a timeless, asocial, indeed, *pre*-social existence of dispassionate ignorance. And the idea of society which emerges from this self is one, if not actually chosen, capable of being chosen, and therefore a product of the individual will. The view of justice which results from these starting points is thereby a derivative of the moral will of autonomous individual agents, a social ethics which arises from the requirements imposed by an atomistic moral anthropology. Finally, the Rawlsian view of justice, like other liberal, contractarian views, is the after-thought of an essentially complete individualistic morality, a chosen compromise of expedience of singular selves who create society and its properly just, constitutive rules out of their surplus. Thus, neither society nor the just social relationships it embodies contribute to the selfhood of the individuals who form it.

There is a sense, of course, in which we do choose the sort of society we want to live in, at least in democratic states. We choose our leaders, speak out on policies, formulate priorities for social action, and protect individual liberties. Social contract theories are not concerned with this practical level of choices but with the theoretical underpinning which can justify social arrangements in general. The liberal contractarian assumpiton is that individuals *choose* to live in a society at all, and it is this choice, to be social rather than live as singular individuals, that concerns them. The idea that this can be a choice and that the mode of conceiving justice is an off-spring of individual moral sovereignty is the problem. To see how deeply this is written into our character we should look at another liberal contractarian, John Locke.

Locke's *Second Treatise of Government* (1690) is arguably the most important document in support of the liberal constitutional state. Written as a rationale for resistance to Charles II in the battle over succession to the English throne, it became a vindication of the Glorious Revolution of 1688 and, nearly a century later, an instrument the American colonists turned against British rule.

In contrast to Rawls' original position, Locke begins with persons in a "state of nature," a condition of freedom and equality in which the laws of nature are the guiding norms.[5] In this condition people are entitled to take as their property anything which through their labor they remove from its natural state. In the beginning, Locke says, all the earth "God gave to mankind in common, without any express compact of all the commoners." Private property is carved out of the commons as men mix their labor with nature, thereby altering it and, in Locke's view, making it more productive and useful for all. Appeals to Locke's notion of property frequently fail to consider the qualifications he put on acquisitions. For now, the important point is that labor and property acquisition all occur *before* society is formed. The social compact is, in fact, largely a device to permit the holding and protection of personal property and to safeguard the private sphere.

> Men being, as has been said, by nature, all free, equal, and independent, no one can be put out of this estate, and subjected to the political power of another, without his own consent. The only way whereby any one divests

himself of this natural liberty, and puts on the *bonds of civil society,* is by agreeing with other men to join and unite into a community for their comfortable, safe, and peaceable living one amongst another, in a secure enjoyment of their properties, and a greater security against any, that are not of it.[6]

The beginning and the essence of any political society, Locke maintains, "is nothing but the consent of any number of free men capable of a majority to unite and incorporate into such a society."[7]

The purpose Locke has in mind here is not to articulate a moral individualism but to limit the power of monarchy and support the doctrine of the necessary consent of the governed. Yet even if not the focus of his concerns, the structure of Locke's progression from the individual to the social and the priority of the former is unmistakable. And like Rawls' account, the justice which emerges is one which takes the individual as the most real, indeed, the only real moral element. Society is essentially a human creation, and as it is optional to begin with, it presumably may be dispensed with, as the American of Slater's parable attempted to do.

For Rawls, as Locke before him, the primary act from which justice is derived is an individual act, an assessment of rational self-interest. George Parkin Grant, a Canadian jurist, contrasts the notion of justice in contract liberalism with that to be found in Plato's *Republic.* For Plato, as for most of the ancients, "justice is what we are fitted for."[8] Justice presupposes a view of human beings as normatively structured toward some proper good, the fulfillment of which is to achieve the goal or *telos* of life. Grant points to the vacancy at the heart of modern concepts of justice where only individual self-interest fills the content of the goals of justice and where, therefore, procedural fairness, freedom, and tolerance are thought to be ends in themselves rather than means to a substantive good.[9] We may lament this fact, as Grant does, or praise it, as modern liberals are likely to do, seeing it as liberation from tyrannical notions of the human good which mark traditional societies. The point here is not to judge the lack of content in liberal justice, but to note that such material emptiness and procedural preoccupation is the logical correlate of a concept of the just society which is radically individualistic. Procedural (rather than substantive) justice must flourish where individual liberty is perceived as the primary aim of a just society.

Nozick and Libertarian Justice

Libertarian devotion to moral individualism hardly needs to be argued, for justice here is based on entitlements, "natural rights," and merit and in no way appeals to claims of a common good. Indeed, Robert Nozick, the most eloquent of libertarian theorists, refuses even to accredit the term 'distributive justice' since it begs the issue of the right to distribute. He says, "we are not in the position of children who have been given portions of pie by someone who now makes last minute adjustments to rectify careless cutting. There is no *central* distribution, no person or group entitled to control all the resources, jointly deciding how they are to be doled out."[10] Nozick offers instead the term 'holdings' to signify what individuals have lawfully acquired and to which they are entitled, asserting that if each person's holdings are just, then the distribution must be seen as just also.[11]

In contrast to Rawls' hypothetical contractors in the original position, Nozick offers an entitlement theory which respects historical interactions and transfers. He criticizes Rawls' "end-state principles" of justice as focusing exclusively on outcomes and as blind to how particular distributions of goods and services came about.[12] Contract liberalism, in Nozick's views, always infringes on individual liberties for the sake of society. But 'society' is another term which presumes too much and begs the question Nozick thinks is most important. Pointing out that we as individuals frequently undergo sacrifices for a greater personal good, Nozick asks:

> Why not, *similarly,* hold that some persons have to bear some costs that benefit other persons more, for the sake of the overall social good? But there is no *social entity* with a good that undergoes some sacrifice for its own good. There are only individual people, different individual people, with their own individual lives. Using one of these people for the benefit of others, uses him and benefits the others. Nothing more.[13]

Nozick's response to Rawls is that people in the original position do not have the *right* to decide how everything is to be divided up. Property and entitlements are not "manna from heaven" but belong to individuals as a matter of basic right. Distribution and redistribution, then, always presume doing violence to the integrity of some persons who have prior claims. Thus the minimal state is the only morally defensible or just society.

Rather than argue here with Nozick's conclusions or even his reasoning, our concern is with his beginning points, which for all their differences, he and Rawls share in common. Both begin with assumptions of the plurality and distinctness of persons, or separate existences. Both assume that the task is the *formation* of society, and the task of justice is one of inventing rules by which society will be properly ordered. Rawls' vision of the social order is, of course, more egalitarian and concedes a greater worth to parity of opportunities and prospects among persons, while Nozick rules out redistributive policies altogether. Yet their tacit agreement is more important than their divergent conclusions. For each, social relationships are a choice, an option, and a convenience. Choices to enter a social arrangement presume no previous relatedness, no web of social nurture or sustenance. For both, we are, in our essential nature, isolated selves, on our own, and we may (theoretically for Rawls, actually for Nozick) choose to be social or remain in our individual state of nature.[14]

Thus, the sharpest possible contrasts can be drawn between modern concepts of self and society and ancient ones. Aristotle, for example, claimed that "man is by nature a political animal," or a social creature, and that a person who by nature, and not by accident, is without social lineaments is either a beast or a god, but not a human being. For Aristotle, the gift of speech was itself evidence that man is suited for political life, as man's instincts also tell him. Society is prior to the individual as the whole is prior to one of its parts, and the proof is that "the individual, when isolated, is not self-sufficing."[15]

Modern societies are, of course, a long way from the *polis*, but even granting this, it should be noted that modern conceptions of society are not just different; they are inversions of the Aristotelian ideal. Whereas Aristotle assumes the existence of society and then moves to a consideration of just and virtuous actions of individuals, Rawls and Nozick (as Locke and others before them) assume the existence of individual persons and then proceed to the problem of how to form a just society. For Aristotle, man is by nature social; for moderns, man is by nature (in his "state of nature") solitary and individuated. So what Aristotle would take as the worst possible, even de-humanizing, circumstance for man, modern thought takes as a normative posture. What one view takes as natural and self-evident, the other sees as chosen and in need of regulation and justification.

There is, of course, nothing new in this observation as anyone with a decent course in Western civilization knows. Yet it is worth reminding us that the assumptions made by the leading political theorists of our day are not self-evident and ultimately may not be correct. Every notion of justice rests on basic views of the self and society and their relationship, and Rawls' and Nozick's are no exception. Both are indebted to an individualistic anthropology which cripples their work and provides for only a frail sense of relatedness. To nail down this last point we will need to return to Rawls' concept of community as it is expressed near the end of his book in a section entitled "The Idea of Social Union."

The question is whether contract theory, stressing as it does the individualistic features of fairness, is "a satisfactory framework for understanding the values of community."[16] Rawls presents here two views of community. The first is a purely instrumental association or a "private society" where persons think of social arrangements as necessary burdens and cooperate only because it is necessary to achieve their private aims. Rawls rejects this vision as egoistic and describes his own notion of community as one in which the participants have "shared final ends" and even see cooperation as a good in its own right.[17] Rawls believes this second notion of community is realizable in his scheme because his view of the person does not foreclose on altruism or even personal sacrifice.

Yet even here, the individualism is too pervasive and deep to support anything more than a concept of community as a loose association. Michael Sandel, in a penetrating critique of Rawls, points out that even Rawls' non-egoistic community has no place for an individual whose self-understanding is formed by social ties. Community, he says, describes not just what we *have* as fellow citizens, but what (or better "who") we *are*. Persons who belong to a community see it not as "a relationship they choose (as in a voluntary association) but an attachment they discover, not merely an attribute but a constituent of their identity."[18] Sandel goes on to indicate that an *association* is not a *community*, *reciprocity* does not necessarily make for *sharing*, nor does *cooperation* lead to real *participation* and *attachment*. Rawls' failure to recognize these differences severely hampers his account of justice. As Sandel says, "his theory

of justice depends ultimately for its coherence on precisely
this intersubjective dimension he officially rejects."[19]

Ideal Observer Norms of Justice

Modern ethical theories in general, and theories of justice
in particular, have been concerned with the problem of
reconciling individual self-interest with the desire to live in
a social order where our interests are likely to conflict with
others. One of the favorite ways to attempt such a reconciliation is through recourse to a hypothetical point of
view, an "ideal observer,"[20] who transcends the particulars
of history and culture and achieves an unbiased and universal perspective. The ideal observer embodies a perspective
divested of special interests and at a sufficient distance to
enhance objectivity and remove special pleading. The move
to such a hypothetical chooser satisfies the demand that
ethical judgments be fair (impartial) and consistent (based
on common principles applied uniformly). It also meets
the demand that ethics as a discipline be able to rise above
the fray of self-interested argument and counter-argument
to a level of arbitration and adjudication.

Rawls' "original position" is his technique to accomplish
this ideal observer posture, only he substitutes disinterest
behind the veil of ignorance in his choosers for the traditional formula of omniscience and universal sympathy.[21]
Kant expresses this requirement in terms of the rational
demands of a categorical imperative and universalizability.[22]
Many philosophers believe some such device is an essential
ingredient for ethics, and Kurt Baier goes so far as to equate
the ideal observer perspective with "the moral point of
view."[23]

Rawls believes that the appeal to an ideal observer as
usually conceived tends to make justice utilitarian. So that
if a rightly ordered society is one which an ideal observer

would select, the focus will be on "the net sum of satisfaction" rather than fairness to individuals.[24] Indeed, utilitarian accounts of justice are often posed as alternatives to the individualist emphasis of contractarian views, and some of the most prominent utilitarians, such as David Hume, have made use of some form of ideal observer theory. Yet even here, in the emphasis on the overall or aggregate good, there is an absence of the social dimension, and this cripples the ideal observer as a point from which to perceive justice.

The appeal to an ideal observer, as to contractors in an original position or state of nature, tends to deemphasize the social context in which moral deliberations occur and to which they have reference.[25] This context is always more than a setting or backdrop for choice; it is the locus within which choices live and cohere with the rest of life. The ideal observer is outside of a convivial social order; he is without context and rootless. Social relationships—such as those formed by families, professions, or religious groups—are tangential to the ideal observer. An observer is, by definition, not involved. Involvement entails constraints engendered by fidelity and loyalties to specific others.

The sort of individualism exemplified in the ideal observer is antithetical to communal or social realities altogether. It identifies the paradigm situation of choosing a just society as a posture of disaffiliation and alienation from the social fabric. And this paradigm excludes some essential dimensions of ethics such as past obligations to particular people or responsibilities incurred by familial or professional status.

Generalizability is a necessary criterion for judgments precisely because the paradigmatic situation of choice is that of a person in no social situation in particular. Principles of justice under this scheme are calculated to function as the touchstones of an ethics among strangers. Moral formulae are needed because of the absence of senses of obligation and duty engendered through friendships, families, and communities. In short, in the individualism of ideal observers every judgment must be generally applicable to all because there are presumed to be no morally relevant differences grounded in social life. Hence, it is as rational-agent-to-rational-agent that appeals for fairness and claims to justice are (ideally) made. References to the particulars of persons and communities are, by definition, special appeals and hence biased.

The request to embark upon a process of ideal observing is impossible and pernicious. It is impossible because we are not capable of a God's-eye view. Moreover, moral dispassion is a human pretense. The ideal observer process asks for moral amnesia of a sort that historical creatures are incapable of owning or acting out. It is pernicious because the attempt to emulate an ideal, omniscient perspective tempts us to forsake the moral compass we rightly have—our particular roles as doctor, parent, teacher, and the like. It is in these social roles that moral agents find their orientation and that moral rules find their justification. Indeed, it is only on this basis that we can speak of just or unjust persons, as they exercise their obligations partially or fully, carelessly or faithfully.

Ideal observers choose as a hypothetical omniscient and impartial judge would choose. But there are no omniscient, impartial judges. We could not, in any event, relate to such a judge because there is no agent behind or within the actions that feels as we feel and sees as we see. Such a judge has no place in the human world because such a judge has no history and no personal presence.

A universe in which there is no recourse to the person behind and within the action, a universe in which there is no concrete agent (as opposed to ideal observer) is a universe in which 'good' and 'bad', 'right' and 'wrong', 'just' and 'unjust' have no use. It is precisely into such a universe of moral discourse that ideal observer theory invites us, into a substitution of pseudo-scientific rationality for personal moral integrity. Such an invitation, if taken seriously, would undo ethics entirely. All this is signified by acknowledging that the ideal observer has no proper name; a proper name implies a history, both personal and social, in which a self and other selves are known.

The figure of the ideal observer as portrayed in modern ethical theory is deeply flawed. It ignores some of the most important dimensions of ethics, distorting both social and personal elements. It draws deeply from modern individualism and underestimates the moral force of social roles. Ideal observer norms are probably best understood, not as ideals to be emulated, but as caveats to warn us against vested interests, ignorance, bias, and an impoverished moral imagination. But this essentially negative function cannot carry the weight of the full, positive portrait of justice needed to guide our actions. At most, it can only show us our limitations.

The Absence of the Social

Life in the modern liberal and libertarian state, based on enlightened self-interest, rational calculations, or the norms of an ideal observer, provides only enough social cohesiveness to support a very modest form of social justice. We might eventually develop a sense of belonging if we were lucky enough to have the same goals and life plans as other individuals, but this would inevitably be a thin sense of affinity based on nothing more than expedience and similarity of interests. Shared meaning structures, the ability to see oneself as truly belonging or being a "member" of a society, is not possible because identity and interests are all formed prior to the social contract. Justice in this circumstance will be confined to the *ideal* of respect for persons but without the formative experiences of relatedness that make other persons, or even ourselves, intelligible to us. Without an undergirding and "given" set of experiences which we hold in common, the ideal of respect for the autonomy of others will be empty of content, and civil relationships—including justice—will depend entirely on a grudging respect for a *form* of relationship. Such a society would never enable us to be substantively in touch with the needs of others, for this depends on others becoming more than fellow contractors. In short, the modern society envisioned here gives us no acquaintance with real selves to whom we are bonded, but only generalized others with whom we negotiate. We live and die as aliens, so it is no wonder that remaining in the individual "state of nature" may seem so attractive to some.

Yet the fundamental problem is not that the notions of justice which Rawls, Nozick, or an ideal observer offer us are completely false. All are elegant, forcefully argued positions, and Rawls especially offers much that should be incorporated into our thinking. The real problem is that none of these theories has a sufficient place for the social dimension of life. The sociability of human beings is, of course, recognized by both Rawls and Nozick. Rawls, for example, acknowledges that society is necessary for human life, that social life is a condition for our developing the ability to think and speak, and that even our most self-interested life-plans presuppose a social setting to be actualized.[26] Yet he does not make use of these facts of sociability in his construction of a theory of justice. They are acknowledged but not thought to be theoretically significant or illuminating. So while these authors are not ignorant or unappreciative of the social dimensions, they do not give it sufficient weight in their formulations. Schooled in traditions which are skeptical of all social ties, these authors perpetuate the distinctively American preoccupation with individualism. The just society which results is thereby depleted of the rich and innumerable social supports in which individual liberties and interests can thrive. For individual freedoms and social bonds are not, when properly conceived, opposing but complementary forms of human well-being.

Rawls and Nozick are not so much wrong as irrelevant.

The image of the person they begin with is too finished, too isolated from social forces, too insulated from the passions of fellow creatures. Rawls would likely object that this is a necessary element to secure the consent of individuals to a social order, even if only in principle. But why should we think there is any deep similarity between those behind a veil of ignorance and ourselves constantly immersed in the sea of our social life and institutions? We do not have the luxury (or the limitations) of constructing society from the beginning. Moreover, the effort to begin in this way requires a heavy price—the destruction of just that individual-social dynamic that is inextricably the human situation. Finally, not only Rawls' original position, but the social self which results from it are merely hypothetical. Rawls has forgotten that moral awareness starts in the middle, in the midst of relationships, and the first task is not to reconstruct a mythic beginning but to describe accurately what we find in the present. Getting our present bearings may lessen our anxiety for a beginning we can cognitively control or consent to.

Behind the Rawlsian philosophy is a need to control the origins, to ground the ideal, just society in a beginning we can appreciate rationally. One might well see it, therefore, as another example of great intellectual ingenuity, a system of mental hooks and pulleys by which we try to secure distance from and sovereignty over our social relatedness. But like Slater's American, we achieve it at the cost of distorting our understanding and alienating ourselves from the social ecology which sustains us. Michael Sandel well expresses the outcome of the Rawlsian project: "the sovereign subject is left at sea in the circumstances it was thought to command."[27]

Toward a Recovery of the Social

Our identity as individuals cannot be secured outside of social ties. It is the failure of modern liberal and libertarian views to recognize this that hampers their views of justice and will inevitably distort our perception of how we are related to others. A more correct perception does not deny our individuality, but places it within (rather than prior to) a social context.

The first sign of our sociability is our bodies, for they link us inextricably to a natural succession. As Leon Kass says, "In the navel are one's forebears, in the genitalia our descendants."[28] Modern ethics, nourished in a Cartesian tradition that neglects the body in favor of the thinking subject, is likely also to neglect the historical and social dimensions which come with our bodies. Our bodies, especially as we age, are vivid and sometimes constant reminders that we are not completely autonomous and self-sufficient. What freedom and self-reliance we do achieve is preceded by a long gestation in the womb, both biological and social. Focusing on the body will remind us of this and suggests that any notion of justice which ignores it proceeds at its peril.

It is not just the body in general but several characteristics of our bodies that suit us for social life. The upright posture, for example, brings us face-to-face with others, freeing our hands for shaking (or, no less social, our fists for fighting), and places us at a visual and metaphysical distance from the earth.[29] Speech, to cite another instance, makes sense only within a plurality of speakers—and hearers. In addition there are what Kass terms, "special social passions," such as sympathy, shame, pity, friendliness, gregariousness, esteem, and affability which "permit and are cultivated in community."[30]

On yet another level, to engage in moral argument is a social activity. Moral argument strives to give reasons for our choices and a larger intelligibility to our actions. To give reasons is to affirm tacitly the essentially public and social nature of morality. All moral choices must be in some way capable of public expression and social presence. Giving reasons is an act of seeking community with other moral selves by appealing to their moral sensibilities. In giving reasons we impute moral agency to others, and the justifications offered are designed to elicit a common understanding among us. Moral argument itself, then, refutes a radical individualism and points to moral selves which are at least concerned with persuasion and consensus. This does not argue for sociality, but *presupposes* it.

The point here is that these human characteristics are not simply accidental traits of our nature or incidental to our situation. Rather they define us and mark us as social creatures. An individualism which denies this or attempts to make it a choice of the calculating mind is frankly incoherent. It denies that upon which it relies to make its assertion. Maurice Merleau-Ponty has put it well, claiming that it is one of the tasks of philosophy to help us recover the social world which exists as a permanent though often out-of-focus dimension of existence. While we may reject particular social relationships, we never fail to be situated relative to some form of social existence.

> Our relationship to the social is, like our relationship to the world, deeper than any express perception or any judgment. It is as false to place ourselves in society as an object among other objects, as it is to place society within ourselves as an object of thought, and in both cases the mistake lies in treating the social as an object. We must return to the social with which we are in contact by the mere fact of existing, and which we carry about inseparably with us before any objectification.[31]

The flaw in these theories of justice lies precisely in their effort to "place society within ourselves as an object of thought,"—a thought, a possibility, or an option for the sovereign individual chooser. And while particular social arrangements may, and should, become objects of our critical scrutiny, to make the social dimension of life itself a choice is a *reductio ad absurdum.* The existence of a self which can formulate such a choice is testimony to the social, and forecloses on an individualism which believes it can generate the social *ab original* from its own reason and will. We are in the social world as fish are in water, as a sustaining ecology without which moral life would be impossible. Socrates, though unjustly condemned to death by his fellow citizens, refused to flee Athens because he realized there was no moral life outside the city. What is required is a view of justice that acknowledges this dimension and attends to it as theoretically significant, rather than trivial. A just society cannot neglect the fact of our interdependence in a social world which precedes and nourishes the individualism we so highly prize. Our proclivity to moral individualism is itself a social phenomenon.

Some may feel here an excessive emphasis on the social and believe this leads to an inversion of modern liberal and libertarian philosophies by making the individual derivative from and secondary to social life. For example, Emile Durkheim is usually understood as saying that society exists as a *sui generis* entity prior to and formative of human nature. Individuals are then seen as owing primary allegiance to the society, for whose causes they are deemed expendable. Whether or not this is a correct interpretation of Durkheim, this is not our argument here. Questions of whether societies precede individuals or vice-versa are fruitless chicken-or-egg issues, temporally, ontologically, and morally. The individual and society are complementary rather than competing realities. To deny either or give one a fundamental moral priority or to try to treat them separately would be foolishness. We are not concerned with an argument from an *a priori* notion of "human nature" or from the nature of society, but one based rather on the most elementary and obvious observations about the human condition and our common experiences.

By recalling experiences of our lived world (rather than the hypothetical world of philosophers) and attending carefully to our social ethos we will be able to form more accurate perceptions of our selves, our social life, and the connections between them. There is no knock-down argument to secure these observations against criticism; readers must measure these perceptions against their own. What is offered here is not some proof but an image, a re-visioning that can capture more adequately than individualistic accounts the truth of our situation.

Sympathy

One sign of our sociability is the existence of social passions. Just why any passion might be called "social" is perhaps best explained by recourse to Adam Smith and his notion of sympathy. Frequently associated with the saccharine sentimentality of a drugstore "condolence card," sympathy has a rich philosophical heritage and a much deeper meaning. It is one of the ironies of our situation that the same Scotsman to whom we look for a theoretical vindication of laissez-faire individualism also provides us with one of the most detailed and sophisticated expositions of sympathy. Adam Smith's *Wealth of Nations,* published in 1776, was preceded seventeen years earlier by a neglected but equally important work of moral philosophy, *The Theory of Moral Sentiments* (1759).

"How selfish soever man may be supposed," Smith says, "there are evidently some principles in his nature, which interest him in the fortune of others, and render their happiness necessary to him, though he derives nothing from it, except the pleasure of seeing it."[32] This is the eloquent opening of chapter one, "Of Sympathy," and we need not hold, as he did, a doctrine of human nature to see his point. Smith uses 'sympathy' in the broad sense "to denote our fellow-feeling with any passion whatever."[33] These range from the most trivial to the most profound, and for some Smith offers vivid illustrations. "The mob, when they are gazing at a dancer on the slack rope, naturally writhe and twist and balance their bodies as they see him do, and as they feel that they themselves must do if in his situation."[34]

So, as Smith sees it, sympathy works in the following way: as a sentiment arises in another person, an analogous sentiment springs up in us at the thought of his situation. Sympathy arises not so much from our viewing of another person's passions but from our thought of the situation which excites them as we imaginatively put ourselves in the other person's place. When our brother is on the rack, he says, we do not feel what he feels, but "by the imagination we place ourselves in his situation, we conceive ourselves enduring all the same torments, we enter as it were, into his body, and become in some measure the same person with him, and thence form some idea of his sensations . . . we then tremble and shudder at the thought of what he feels."[35]

Smith's thesis is that sympathy is the origin of moral judgment, the reason why we approve or disapprove of the actions of others. So far from being "merely an emotion" (as opposed to a rational process) or a mutual feeling, for Smith sympathy is that deep sense of praise or blame which accompanies the proper observation of the actions and conditions of others. Rather than, as we are likely to think of it, an involuntary emotion to which we are subject, sympathy is the proper and natural response which marks our human nature and our affinity to each other as human beings. It is contingent upon proper thinking (attentive observation) and the imaginative capacity to put ourselves in another's shoes.

Modern readers are likely to think that Smith is commending sympathy to us, as if to say, "Be sympathetic with others," or "It is good to have sympathy for other people." But to think of sympathy in this way is to misunderstand Smith altogether. For here 'sympathy' is a fact of human nature—not a virtue—and Smith is describing *what* we do and how we are constituted, not what we ought to do. Benevolence and justice, for example, are virtues; sympathy is the capacity which makes them possible.

Our capacity for sympathy does, of course, rise and fall in intensity owing to factors like proximity. It is the role of reason to render our sentiments more public and social —to extend them beyond the range of our immediate encounters. To do this, principles of moral reasoning are required, and this will be the focus of chapter four. For now the key insight is that even a sympathy restricted to direct experience bespeaks a moral sensibility which is social at its roots.

Sympathy works in our moral judgments of ourselves through our ability to judge our own behavior as if it were someone else's, through the eyes of the "impartial spectator." But unlike the device of the "ideal observer," Smith's "impartial spectator" is not tainted by an individualistic character. The spectator is a way of appropriating a social relatedness, of admitting into account the common moral sentiments of a community. Smith never seems to have had in mind an omniscient vantage-point removed from social ties and personal loyalties. In fact, the impartial spectator is a part of the move of imaginative sympathy so central to Smith's notion of moral judgment.

The ideal observer serves as a device for evoking a model of hypothetical choice, a model which is removed from and above the social fabric. The impartial spectator, by contrast, serves as a way of evoking an alternative or counterbalance in actual choices, a mirror which carries the larger social sentiment and is roughly synonymous with social conscience. As Smith says, "This is the only looking-glass by which we can, in some measure *with the eyes of other people* scrutinize the propriety of our own conduct."[36]

As Raphael and Macfie indicate, the impartial spectator is not a vague, generalized social other, but what anyone would feel if he were a spectator to his own actions, informed with a social conscience.[37] It represents an internal dialectic between personal self-interest and a socially formed perception of the good. The move is not one of displacement from current partiality, but inclusion of the partiality of others as they might view the action. The impartial spectator attempts to appropriate the moral horizon of others, while the ideal observer dispenses with any moral horizon whatever. The impartial spectator is a robust character of social importance in the agent's internal moral dialogue.

It could be objected at this point that sympathy is an inadequate guide for our moral judgments and that moral reasoning must be founded on something more substantial than sentiment. For example, Elmer Sprague claims that Smith makes sympathy an absolute "without considering whether someone might sympathize with 'wrong' affections."[38] Yet this criticism misses the point. Smith's account of our moral sentiments is not intended as a justification of a *principle* of sympathy. It is not an effort to claim that our sentiments are incorrigible, or always morally correct, or to ground all moral reasoning in sentiment. To attribute these agendas to Smith is to read him as a twentieth-century, analytic, moral philosopher rather than for what he is, which is a keen observer of what we might now refer to as moral psychology or social anthropology. In the *Moral Sentiments,* a very long treatise, Smith gives only passing thought near the end to arguments against those who want to base morality in utility or egoism. Smith's aim is not to justify some moral principle or rule, such as benevolence or altruism, against the moral skeptic or egoist, but to describe what he believes we would all, upon reflection, recognize.

Smith's importance for us lies in the power of his descriptions of how we are affected and respond to the situations of others and the way in which we come to judge ourselves. The key insight is that the range and depth of our sympathy is inalienably tied to our social existence.

Sympathy, the seat of morality for Smith, does not depend on conscious acts of will, rational assessments of harm or benefit, noble purposes, charity, good will, or altruism. It is simply part of the human condition that we are sympathetic beings, and it is on this uncalculated and unwilled responsiveness that morality depends. Moral sentiments, to be sure, must be educated and refined, and they are no guarantee against mistakes. But unlike Rawls and Nozick, who begin with abstract, universal traits of self-interest and rationality for human beings, Smith recognizes the presence of a social sentiment as a human endowment essential to our self-understanding.

Smith's emphasis on the moral sentiments issues is a view of self and society that is markedly different than those we have previously examined. In the section "Justice and Beneficence," he says man is "fitted by nature" for social life, and "has a natural love for society, and desires that the union of mankind should be preserved for its own sake, and though he himself was to derive no benefit from it. The orderly and flourishing state of society is agreeable to him, and he takes delight in contemplating it."[39]

The claim that human beings are inextricably social does not deny the existence or power of self-interested motives, nor that private self-interests are frequently in conflict with public-spirited social sentiments. To deny either self-interested sentiments or social sentiments would belie the facts. The point is that all our moral sentiments, even the most egoistic, are rooted in a social ethos and cannot be taken out of it and made to stand alone. Both Rawls and Nozick offer us an anthropology in which self-interest logically precedes a social environment, and they neglect the philosophical import of particular social passions altogether. The British moral philosophers of the eighteenth century were wiser, recognizing the presence of both self-interested and social forces within us.[40]

To claim that human beings have social passions or, like Smith, to claim that moral judgments have their source in sympathy does not argue for a particular view of the just society. Rather it clears the ground on which arguments can be built and designates the moral sense to which arguments can appeal. The individualistic assumptions with which many theories of justice begin are untenable. They are distorted perceptions of both self and society. Their efforts to secure a solid basis for consent to social relatedness and subsequent individual liberties are bought at the price of jeopardizing social relatedness altogether. It is impossible to see how individuals, beginning to form a social order out of only rational self-interest, could ever belong to any society at all. These assumptions fail entirely to acknowledge the extent to which we are social, like it or not, as well as overlook the extent to which our ability to judge our self-interest is socially grounded.

Adam Smith is not the only one to have noted this aspect of our moral perceptions. Both David Hume and Bishop Butler are worth careful study on this point. Smith's moral philosophy is simply one of the most eloquent and richly laced. In contemporary social psychology one could point to the work of George Herbert Mead and Harry Stack Sullivan, among others, as congenial to the inherently social existence of the self. Martin Buber's poetic expression of the I-Thou and I-It relationships as prior to any atomic sense of self, with an ontological and moral primordiality, is a religious instance of this mode of thinking. And H. Richard Niebuhr's response ethics is a notable instance of the sort of reasoning to be commended as the basis of justice. Niebuhr sought to overcome the limitations both of traditional teleological ethics, which perceives a person's primary relationship as to 'the good', and of traditional deontological ethics, which places persons first and foremost before the moral law or duty. Niebuhr's alternative was what he called a response ethics. Niebuhr found the ethics of response the most adequate to describe biblical traditions, and the most realistic in its assessment of the human situation. A response ethics, says Niebuhr, acknowledges the reality of prior action toward the self, so that ethics is, fundamentally, being responsive to (and responsible for) the others to whom one is in relationship. A response ethics calls our attention to "the fundamentally social character of selfhood."[41] By this Niebuhr means that not only do we come to know ourselves only in relationships, but that we exist as moral selves only in relationships.

> To say the self is social is not to say that it finds itself in need of fellow men in order to achieve its purposes, but that it is born in the web of society as a sentient, thinking, needful being with certain definitions of its needs and with the possibility of experience of a common world. It is born in society as mind and as moral being, but above all it is born in society as self.[42]

Moral arguments always appeal to, and presuppose, a certain moral sense. This moral sense cannot be argued for, but only toward, or evoked as the backdrop or tacit sense of reality which provides a touchstone for the principles. To argue for the moral sense which undergirds the arguments for principles is to beg the question of presupposing the priority in our sensibility of that which we want to prove. The social sense of self is a given within experiences and perceptions which we can deny only with great difficulty and at the cost of coherence. Whatever principles of justice we espouse must acknowledge and affirm what Louis Dumont calls "the apperception of the social nature of man."[43] We have an innate sympathy with others and a susceptibility to the pleasures of human association. Sympathy provides the capability, and sentiments supply the affective basis of justice, but neither provide an adequate or full expression.

Principles are necessary in order to discern the scope of application of these sentiments, to overcome the debilitating effects of "moral distance," to discipline and order our social passions and direct them appropriately. But even here, before the regulating and extending power of principles come into play, these moral sentiments both imply and require a social setting which constitutes our moral life and is not just tangential to it. So even here we are beyond the superficial renderings of the Good Samaritan story as either the largesse or reflexive sentimentality of individuals. Rather the story is revelatory of the basic relatedness of all human life.

The perception of the Samaritan was of a fellow human being, a neighbor, and his virtue lay not only in the helping acts he performed but in the perception that he was of one fabric with the beaten man in the road. He had compassion, we are told, a term which literally denotes, "to suffer with." Thus Adam Smith's 'sympathy' and the Samaritan's compassion point us in a common direction and designate a primal recognition of self in our perception of others. This is the fundamental grounding for all principles and theories of justice, in the absence of which no reasoning, calculations, prudence, or philanthropy will have a motive force. In the needs of others we see ourselves, recognize our own neediness, and acknowledge our own vulnerability.

Yet even this recognition, basic though it is, does not tell us how to choose when there are multiple victims in the road. And though circumstances of proximity will undoubtedly lead us naturally to extend our sympathy to some more than others, it is not self-evident that ties of proximity in age, sex, status, or blood are reliable guides for our choices. The simple solution (but not necessarily the most just) is to help those who are immediately before us while refusing to admit that we have made a choice at all. This is to choose by default, as we now practice a rationing by default to an economic model of medicine. Principles are required to shape and make feasible, as well as to sharpen our perceptions of justice, and to be responsible for, as well as responsive to, our social sentiments.

4. Principles of Justice: Rights and Needs

A sense of ourselves as social creatures is a beginning, but it is not sufficient. So far the arguments have been largely negative—ruling out certain individualistic concepts of self and society—and illustrative—in the sense of pointing and appealing to a sense of moral selfhood that is socially grounded. At best, these observations can orient our thinking, but they do not make the case for any policy of distributive justice. To do this principled argument is required to show why we should accept some principles of justice over others as we ration health care resources. Perceptions of justice without principles are like blind motives or good intentions without a sense of direction. Principles of justice which are not grounded in perceptions and moral sensibilities are empty formalisms. Affirming principles will deepen our perceptions, just as perceptions will be honed through their expression as principles.

Rights Language: Problems and Prospects

Sooner or later all considerations of justice in health care must consider the question of whether health care is a right, and if so, what that means. Rights language has become the favored way to address the issue, and this is hardly surprising, for all of our moral language seems to have been taken over by this idiom. In the recent past all proponents of social change have employed rights rhetoric to couch their claims. Civil rights, women's rights, and gay rights have been some of the most visible instances, but the extension of such claims has reached a considerable distance into health care as well. The Hospital Patients' "Bill of Rights," the rights of children, of psychiatric patients, of those who refuse treatment, and of the dying are examples but do not exhaust the list. Physicians have claimed their rights as well, most notably the right to choose whom they will serve. So it is not surprising that in this atmosphere of a banquet of rights, the right to health care should become the focus of questions about justice.

This obsession with rights language is unfortunate, primarily because it feeds the individual and private notion of self. In many instances those who claim rights neglect its rich, moral legacy in favor of a notion of rights as quasi-legal absolutes. Holders of rights are frequently conceived as having overriding claims, to which no opposition or abridgment can be tolerated. Too often, as in the abortion debate, rights claims are thought to have such a preeminence over all other moral considerations that to wield a right is to apply the *coup de grace* in moral argument. Some (though not all) feminists claim total "reproductive rights," while "pro-lifers" put forward a "right-to-life" for the unborn. Both seem to be acting on the assumption that they hold unassailable ground.

Ronald Dworkin captures the tone of such rhetoric nicely in calling rights "political trumps held by individuals."[1] In the current climate rights seem to function as truncheons. In either case, rights have taken on an absolutist flavor and are tools of moral debate (or castigation) wielded by individuals as claims against others. Recourse to an individualized and absolute notion of rights is frequently used as a conversation-stopper and as an excuse against further probing. The idea of rights as trumps held by individuals is only one dimension of the moral significance of rights. When taken by itself it distorts other key notions of social life, such as responsibility, and more generally, the role of the person in a larger communal order of living.

The reason why rights language has lost its deeper social reference is, of course, easy to see in the legacy bequeathed to us from political philosophies and cultural traditions. An ethos of individualism which is innately skeptical about, and believes it has sovereignty over, social relationships dovetails with a notion of rights as negative absolutes— immunities from interference by others and defenses of individual liberties and entitlements. What is needed is a notion of rights that incorporates individual liberties with a lively sense of social interdependence.

While it is true that rights, when inscribed into law, can and do entail specific claims and duties, the moral notion of rights is more complex. Neglect of this complexity cripples the debate about a right to health care.

For H. L. A. Hart, a moral right is something to be taken into account, not an obligation to undertake or refrain from a specific action.[2] Joel Feinberg says that rights are the grounds of obligation.[3] Rights do generally imply correlative duties, yet it would be naive to think that the mere assertion of a right somehow settles an issue like access to health care. Ascribing rights is only a first step in moral discernment; a second and necessary step is deciding what ascribing rights to persons amounts to and what actions, if any, licitly follow.

Rights are never conclusive until their range of application is specified. The task is to delineate carefully the scope of a right as it is brought into play in particular instances. This is precisely what is foreclosed by the absolutist doctrine of rights.

To say that rights are not absolutes is not to say that rights are relative or that they can be upheld only when it seems convenient. Indeed, the allegation of relativism simply misses the point. Absolutist and relativist doctrines of rights both presuppose a private and possessive individualism.

Rights are also distorted if they are treated as private possessions. The claim "I have a right to . . ." is often thought to be a claim of a sovereignty over a range of choice and action. Such an interpretation is adversarial and anti-communal, precisely because conflicting absolute claims do not acknowledge, and tend to erode, the social foundations on which any rights claim can be made.

The claim "I have a right to do X" stated absolutely indicates a need for moral certainty, that is, the need to guarantee the rightness of a choice in advance and irrespective of context and history. Doing "X" may, of course, turn out to be good or evil, but it is—on this reading—one to which *I* am entitled and in this way, a choice beyond reproach. Such purity and security of choice, however, is a manipulation of individual prerogatives beyond any common sense of morality.

The Social Ethos of Rights

Personal rights and social interdependence are inseparable aspects of human life. Individual freedom is a social reality. Individual rights are rooted in a social reality that antedates them and gives them meaning. Each of us can exercise rights in a meaningful way only so long as these rights are recognized and respected by others. Rights are social in the sense that a social context must exist for them to have any meaningful range of application. But the social meaning of rights has a deeper sense.

Rights for individuals make sense at all only within a social ethos. Just as there is no freedom without a field of action, there are no individual rights outside a social ambiance. A convivial order is the condition for the possibility of a rights claim. Assertions of rights are claims for

recognition within the moral commons. Acknowledgment
of rights claims are recognition that others are also members of the commons. Every notion of natural or human
rights implies mutuality within a social order, that is, the
recognition of others who are equals in moral prerogative
and agency.

The social ethos of rights indicates that rights claims are
ways of displaying our humanity. Rights define us, delineate our moral agency, symbolize our mutual self-regard.
Natural or human rights apply to persons irrespective of
class, economic condition, race, religion, or other contingent conditions. Such rights are anterior to particular social
contracts and are not abolished by political revolutions
because they are based in a social sense of self that antedates formal governments and institutions. Indeed, in
Western democracies, governments are thought to derive
their just powers from their fidelity to a more primordial
social order in which the rights of all individuals are
respected.

Natural or human rights are, therefore, not individual
but social in character, or better, individual only because
they are social. The social dimension is not a human creation constituted by choice for the convenience of individuals, nor is it merely an aggregate of individuals. Sociality
is a given and inalienable state of affairs. We are innately
social, not social by choice, and rights are one expression
of the meaning of our sociality.

The human being is individual and social. Acknowledging
this deep reciprocity between the individual and the social
dimensions of human life supports neither individualism
nor socialism as political ideologies. Rather it indicates the
need for a sense of morality in which individual rights and
social obligations are seen as mutually critical and interpretive dimensions of a single moral phenomenon.

It is the institutions and roles of social life that give to
individual rights their purpose and completeness. Without
our social lineaments, rights are empty formalisms, lacking

a historical context or a political meaning. The choice between individual rights and social obligations is not one between conflicting alternatives but between complementary dimensions. Neither makes sense without the other. If the social ethos of rights is neglected, moral disputes will continue to be jousting matches for individual superiority in an antagonistic commons.

There is a right to health care, but it is a right which must be carefully defined within, and responsive to, the social ambiance. This refinement must wait, however, until we have examined the claims of those who deny that there is such a right at all.

The Right to Health Care vs. Prior Rights

Acknowledging the social character of rights points to the difficulties in Robert Nozick's denial of a right to health care. Libertarians such as Nozick are fond of the notion of "rights as trumps held by individuals" because they believe that any scheme of distributive justice wrongly presupposes allocative prerogatives and violates individuals' entitlements to their holdings. In *Anarchy, State and Utopia,* Nozick compares doctors to barbers, claiming that there is no more reason to distribute doctors according to need than to distribute barbers according to need.[4] In both cases the redistribution would do violence to the prior claims doctors and barbers have to control their own actions. We may believe that because doctors perform a more socially valued service that we can control their actions, but Nozick asserts that doctors, just like anyone else, have a prior right of entitlement.

The flaw in his argument is, again, to view rights from an individualistic and not a social perspective. The fatal move is to assume at the outset that entitlement rights exist logically prior to (and, in the state-of-nature hypothetical schema, historically prior to) the existence of society, so that the social order can be viewed as having emerged out of a wish to protect the rights that people have in the state of nature and that they bring with them into the social compact. But this is like saying that trumps existed prior to the game of bridge, and that from some earlier state, the game of bridge evolved because people had these trumps lying around. Here bridge is just the (dispensable) occasion to use trumps. The analogy drives home the point that rights exist, and have both meaning and substance, only if one presupposes a social context, just as trumps make no sense outside of bridge.[5]

An argument similar to Nozick's, but couched more in terms of laissez-faire economics, is made by Robert Sade. In a well-known article in the *New England Journal of Medicine* in 1972, Sade claims that there is no right to health care. His position is that since a physician owns his professional skills, he is entitled to dispense with them as he pleases. As bread belongs to the baker who made it, to sell at whatever price he wishes, so medical services belong to the physician. To force the physician into a fee schedule or to oblige him to see patients he does not choose or make him a government employee (in, say, a National Health Service) is to violate the physician's liberty and his right to practice as he sees fit.[6]

Sade believes that justice is served when the free market is preserved because the market is the least restrictive and most respectful of individual rights. So if a physician chooses to serve those who cannot pay, it is a charitable act, but not one which is in any sense obligated. The patient has no right to care, but can purchase it if he or she is able.

Critics of the laissez-faire model of justice, or "market justice"[7] argue that it is flawed in three ways:[8]

The first flaw is that persons are not in a bargaining position when they are ill or injured. Persons seek a physician when they are compromised—functionally, physically, and psychologically. They are therefore not free, rational agents in the market, able to barter and choose intelligently among the services available to them.

Seeking help when one is ill is not like shopping for a shirt or soliciting bids on a building project. The "sick role" entails a somewhat compromised capacity to judge, and it includes a restriction on what is optimally only a theoretical range of choices about whom to see and how much to pay for services. A free market for medicine could not protect patients from the minority of physicians (or their corporate employers) who would prey on the sick for personal profit (or corporate survival). The patient as free agent is largely a fiction.

The second flaw in the market model of justice is the idea that physicians constitute a supply and demand market. The classic laws of supply and demand do not operate in medical care. The evidence shows that just the reverse occurs. The greater the supply of physicians, the greater the demands and the greater the cost for medical services. This is so because physicians largely generate their own business. They are simultaneously the experts who decide *who needs care, how much care, and what kind of care* patients need (gatekeepers), and the recipients of the financial rewards. This dual role provides no incentives for cost control and exacerbates the market difficulties. Moreover, physicians are largely bound to each other by non-competitive, fraternal ties, exemplified in the traditional prohibition of advertising.

The third argument against market justice is that it contains a tacit and unacceptable merit criterion for access to care. "To each according to ability to pay" functions on the (largely unspoken) premise that those who can afford health services are deserving, while those who cannot afford them may not be. While the poor are rarely explicitly said to be unworthy of care, tacit negative assumptions about the indigent are correlate of letting market forces dictate access. (Consider recent debates about just who constitutes the "deserving" poor.) Market justice rewards those with financial resources and disenfranchises further those who lack such resources. Market justice follows, and accepts as normative, the economic disparities that already exist in society. Market justice says that disparities of wealth can legitimately translate into disparities of health care. It sees the financial barriers to health care as unfortunate, but not unfair.

Thus there are a number of problems underlying the market model for health care which disqualify it as the primary principle of distribution. Yet the fundamental problem is not with the market *per se,* but with the individualism of Sade's vision of the market. The market can be adjusted to accommodate the objections raised against it; by providing advisors and education for patients, by changing incentives for cost control, and/or by providing funds for the poor to enter the medical market. Some of these measures have been tried, with modest results. But none of these adjustments would change the fundamental individualism that underlies Sade's position. For his basic commitments are not to the market as a distributional device, but to a concept of rights. The core notion is, like Nozick's, one of private entitlements, garnered anterior to any social relationship, and without obligation, which it is the primary duty of society to protect. But, as we have seen, this image of self and society is gravely distorted. And this is no less true of physicians than for others in society. In fact, the doctor's route for coming into possession of and exercising his or her skills is far more socially supported than other positions or professions.

For example, over half the cost of medical education and about forty percent of the cost of health care services are paid out of public funds.[9] This does not close the case, as Victor Sidel believes, in favor of a right to health care, but it does at least move us beyond a naive notion of Lockean ownership of professional skills. Physicians do not acquire their knowledge and skills or apply them by independently realized labor from a state of nature. Older traditions of professionalism are clear on this, seeing the holding of expert skills not as a piece of private property but as a public trust.[10] The religious term for this is 'stewardship'. But even outside of religious contexts, professionals have borrowed the religious language of fiduciary relationships to express their status and press their claims.

James Childress correctly points out that although physicians in training and in practice accept public funds, there is no explicit contract, nor even an explicit expectation of obligation, at the time the funds are offered and accepted. Indeed, many medical students are, no doubt, unaware of this assistance. Childress argues, therefore, that there should be considerable discretion about how any such obligation to the public should be met.[11] But Sade's premises are fictional for, in Nozick's words, we must look not only to allocation outcomes but to "where the things or actions to be allocated and distributed come from."[12] And at least a *prima facie* case can be made, on Nozick's own terms—on the basis of historical entitlements—for turning a portion of physicians' skills toward the public which helped them acquire those skills.

A variety of other measures by which health professionals are supported by public actions and assisted by regulations could also be discussed here—licensing laws, accreditation practices, and other means by which the professional mandate is vested in providers because of the public good that is thought to accrue. Traditionally, professional self-regulation has been given to medicine in exchange for services society needs and values. All of these are ways in which physicians, both individually and collectively, profess to be a part of the larger social order.

This is not to say that health professionals have no rights, or that there may not be times when the rights of individual practitioners need to be asserted against the inflated expectations and demands of individual patients

or a dubious agenda of the state. The efforts to enlist physicians in the execution of criminals or in some military
operations may be legitimate occasions for physicians to
protect their professional integrity by evocation of prior
rights of refusal or non-involvement. But here the appeal
to prior rights is grounded simply in different sets of social
obligations rather than individual entitlements. Prior rights
always imply a social context, and while this recognition
does not make the case for a right to health care, it removes
the libertarian impediments frequently erected against it.

The Right to Health Care vs. Freedom

A position in some ways similar to Nozick's but with
greater stress on freedom is that of H. Tristram Engelhardt.
He begins with an assumption of society as secular and
pluralistic, in which a variety of different communities
must peaceably resolve their differences. Such a society, he
argues, will be unwilling to impose on its diverse citizenry
a single concept of the good life and will tolerate the freedom of its members to pursue their own goals as they see
fit with minimal interference, so long as the similar freedoms of others are not abridged.[13] This tolerance and freedom must also mark definitions of health and health care,
so that "rights to health care are more created than discovered," owing to pluralistic definitions of health itself.[14]
There is, Engelhardt claims, no morally compelling reason
for any particular health care system. Such a system cannot be discovered in the nature of persons, their association,
or in the practices of medicine. All these are culturally relative, subject to human priorities and perceptions of what
is valuable, and contingent across time and space. So whatever health care system and health priorities are devised
must be created by the will of the moral communities
which compose society. The only constraint is the minimal

condition necessary for moral dialogue—respect for the freedom of others.[15] All else is based on aesthetic choice, emotional preference, custom, etc., but not on anything inherent in the nature of things. Thus, in Engelhardt's view, a society could decide to spend all its health resources on rhinoplasty and hip reductions and neglect cancer research or infectious diseases, and this may seem an odd set of priorities, but it would not be necessarily wrong. Moreover, health care could be ignored altogether. "The choice of art over health care may, thus, be a bizarre, but not an intrinsically immoral choice."[16] Why? Because "the provision for health care, unlike respect for the freedom of moral agents, is not essential for the possibility of the moral life."[17]

The result is that rights to health care, unless derived from a special contractual agreement, depend on the principle of beneficence, and therefore, are likely to conflict with the stronger principle of autonomy. So like Nozick, Engelhardt's version of self and society begins with the assumption that whatever resources exist are private, rather than common. Inequities in these resources, so that the wealthy, the well-placed, those with media-appeal, or good insurance get, say, liver transplants while others do not, are "unfortunate but not unfair."[18] In sum, there is no right to have corrections made for, or protections against, the exigencies of the natural or social lottery.

In his new book *The Foundations of Bioethics,* Engelhardt discusses what he takes to be the root tension at the heart of ethics between autonomy and beneficence. Autonomy is more basic, he claims, because beneficence is always contingent on some notion of the good, and ultimately, definitions of the good have to be agreed upon commonly and freely. So "the principle of beneficence is exhortatory, while the principle of autonomy is constitutive."[19] It is for this reason that Engelhardt prefers Nozick over Rawls. Nozick embodies what he calls a freedom-based system of justice which sets limits to the goals a society can pursue constrained by freedom and property rights, while Rawls espouses a goal-based system of justice which presumes to define the desirable outcomes in advance.[20]

Several objections can be raised to Engelhardt's view of the person, of health, and of social life. To some extent his assumptions about the relationship between the self and society mirror those of Nozick, Rawls, Locke, and others. Like his predecessors, he has no place for a moral self which is constitutively formed by life in a social world. Although he does accredit life in particularistic communities as valid, he does not seem to lend theoretical weight to this fact. It is worth noting that advocacy for individualism is frequently connected with a conviction that freedom, or autonomy, is the highest value, and, in liberalism, the notion that tolerance is the greatest virtue. The pairing of autonomy with beneficence as the root tension of ethics indicates that the freedom denoted here is largely a negative one which sees coercion as the greatest evil, even for beneficent ends. In a universe devoid of intrinsic notions of right and wrong or good and evil, freedom becomes not only the greatest value but the condition of all other values.

Objection could also be made to Engelhardt's relativism, and Leon Kass, among others, has done much to persuade us that nature (hence disease, health, well-being) is not just what we choose. But to dwell on this would distract us from the major points on which Engelhardt's thesis runs aground: (1) that freedom is itself contingent in many cases upon the provision of health care, and (2) that the structure of social life contributes heavily to the differences which mark the natural lottery.

(1). The relationship between freedom and access to health care is of great importance, potentially for many of us, and actually for some of us. Most considerations of distributive justice highlight the *tension* between liberty and equitable access to needed care. Providing equitable care for all in need will invariably restrict the liberties of some (notably physicians and other health professionals) and a granting of maximal liberty (to physicians) is not conducive to meeting a goal of equitable access (for patients). This is a standard interpretation of the problem and one which Engelhardt shares.

While this tension is real, to focus on it exclusively as *the* problem of justice overlooks a more fundamental relationship between access to health care and freedom. Harold Laski, in a quote attributed to L. T. Hobbhouse, said "Liberty without equality is a name of noble sound and squalid result."[21] A liberty which does not recognize the material conditions necessary for liberty is as good as no liberty at all. My freedom is empty if my disease or disability prevents me from acting, or forecloses the real possibility of choosing from the start.

Freedom as a goal requires a minimal level of health care as a means. To the extent that we value the freedom of others, to that extent we must be committed to access to the health care necessary to achieve their freedom. Otherwise a commitment to their freedom is empty. Any moral system which values autonomy over beneficence must also realize that beneficence is sometimes necessary to achieve autonomy. Our ability to act as relatively free and independent agents is contingent upon a vast array of previous beneficent acts toward us that supported and nurtured our achievement of that autonomy.

So while at one level of analysis, liberty and equity are at odds, at a more primitive level of human functioning, liberty (in any meaningful sense) is dependent upon a range of action and reflection only possible for the healthy, or those who are reasonably confident that their ill health, present or anticipated, will not become a barrier to their life-plans. For many people in this country the choice to seek medical attention is bought at the price of sacrifice of another of life's necessities. This is a poor freedom indeed, a caricature of liberty, which not only makes liberty the supreme value but also makes it merely an abstract ideal.

Thus, the problem here is the notion that freedom is a natural state which requires little or nothing to be realized.

In reality when we are hungry, hurt, or disenfranchized we realize how radically contingent and fragile our freedom is and how interdependent we are on others to help us achieve and maintain our personal autonomy.

We can agree with Engelhardt that autonomy is a high value, in the absence of which other goods of life are diminished in meaning, but focusing on the tension between autonomy and the beneficence meeting of needs will distort and confine the notion of autonomy too severely. Autonomy is more an achievement of just communities than a given or natural condition of individuals.

We will finally have to choose between limiting the freedom of some or undermining the *conditions* of freedom for others, and this is, to be sure, not a simple choice. If the sick poor are to have freedom at all, some freedoms of health professionals will have to be bounded. But to leave it at this is fundamentally to misunderstand the point. An unlimited, individual freedom is a mistaken concept to begin with and not a right anyone can claim. Moreover, freedom can be served in a variety of ways. It is not self-evident, even from a conviction that autonomy is the prime value in the moral life, that beneficence and equity take a back seat. For our values reside, not in independence from each other in some hierarchical ranking, but in a moral symbiosis. Libertarians are fond of pointing out that a secure life marked by lack of personal freedom is not worth having. But they neglect the converse of this, that a personal liberty or autonomous life is not even possible when physical necessity reduces our choices to the meager and brutal options of a Hobbesian survival ethics. To claim that we prize and protect the freedoms of the disenfranchized while failing to act materially for the welfare which would provide their freedom is naive at best.

(2). The structure of social life frequently exacerbates, and sometimes even causes, differences in the natural lottery. Fifty years ago Henry Sigerist claimed "the chief cause of disease is poverty."[22] Research on the relationship between race, class, poverty, and health consistently shows the same pattern. Economic and social conditions play a role not only in health care, but in overall health. Some are in ill health because they are poor; some are poor because they are in ill health. Most researchers assume that the effects of poor health and low socioeconomic status are circular. Whatever the precise relationship, it is sufficiently clear that class differences contribute to the etiology of disease, so that disease is not just a natural component of the human genetic lottery, not just a chance and uncontrollable occurrence for which no one is responsible. George Silver puts it graphically:

> The air we breathe, the water we drink, the food we eat are poisoned, contaminated with carcinogens and heavily pathogenic, so that we all suffer the consequences. But not equally. The poor live in areas of cities where air is dirtier and concentration of lead is greater, so children of the poor are poisoned more quickly than suburban children. The water of the poor is piped from foul faucets in decaying slum dwellings where typhoid and salmonella thrive.... Factor workers, not the managerial and executive class, are the ones exposed to poisons and hazards and carcinogens of the ill-protected workers.[23]

The idea of a natural lottery (the phrase is Rawls') is one which obscures social complicity in disease occurrence and fits nicely with an individualism which considers persons as essentially complete in the state of nature. If all disease can be attributed to original patterns in the genetic pool, rather than to our historical existence in social patterns, then all obligations to alter or be responsive to these social patterns are optional and gratuitous responses of charity. The 'natural lottery' concept functions here to reinforce the myth of innocence and disclaimers of responsibility. If social class has nothing to do with disease and health, we can say that inequities in access to health care are unfortunate, but not unfair. But this is not the case.

All diseases are not socially determined, but the social structure in which we live plays a part in if, when, how often, and with what malady we fall ill. Not all our health problems relate to social conditions, but, more than it is comfortable to think about, many of them do. So we cannot agree with Englehardt's conclusion that "the differences in need, both medical and financial, must be recognized as unfortunate . . . but not unfair."[24] Sometimes the unfairness results precisely from our participation in the social nexus which contributed to those differences, both medical and financial. The natural lottery turns out to be not so natural as it appeared.

For all there is to admire in Engelhardt's espousal of freedom, it finally does not serve us well. Emphasizing the theoretical conditions for moral agency rather than the material conditions for real choice, Engelhardt defines autonomy too narrowly. A more fulsome view should recognize the social involvement in the distribution of ill health. These dimensions must inform our thinking about a right to health care. While rights claims restrict the freedoms of some, they are materially necessary to the freedom of others. But the argument should not be over freedom vs. some other value, but degrees of freedom, and the meaning of freedom. The individualist, atomic freedom claimed by Nozick, Sade, and Engelhardt does not accurately reflect the human situation and is untenable as a premise. The basic temptation is to suppose that individual freedom is "for free," without cost or effort, and not a goal which communities and just societies must achieve for their members through strenuous efforts. Getting past that sort of naiveté is essential to thinking about justice in health care.

The Right to Health Care vs. Individual Responsibilities

Some objections to a right to health care are pragmatic rather than theoretical. These objections are based on observations of health behaviors and worries about the practical consequences of enacting a right to health care.

One such objection can be called the "merit argument." It goes something like this. Most of the illnesses that occur today are ones which persons inflict upon themselves. Smoking, excessive alcohol consumption, overeating, high cholesterol, and low fiber diets are only the chief examples. Driving without seat belts, hang gliding, motorbike racing, and sexual promiscuity are additional examples of "lifestyle" practices which are productive of disease and disability. The diseases which result—lung cancer, emphysema, cirrhosis of the liver, coronary artery disease, gastrointestinal cancers, automobile injuries and fatalities, and a variety of sexually transmitted afflictions—are all caused, at least in part, by choices to live in an unhealthy way. Such diseases account for over seventy percent of all morbidity and mortality and a great majority of health care expenditures. To grant a right to health care is, therefore, unjustified. Rights imply responsibilities, and many persons in our culture seem loath to live responsibly in terms of avoiding practices they know to be conducive to early death and disability. In such a climate, a right to health care is both undeserved and impractical.

This argument has considerable appeal. A vast number of disabilities, illnesses, and deaths—due to causes not always beyond our control—do occur each year. In view of this evidence, people do have an effect on—and therefore a responsibility for—their own medical needs. Insofar as lifestyles influence mortality and morbidity, there is substantial force in the merit argument for medical care distribution. But to stop here would oversimplify the process of assigning responsibility as well as overestimate our ability to identify causes. We now recognize that the causes of illness are multiple, and their lines of influence and interaction very complex. Also, there remains a broad range of natural contingencies over which we have neither voluntary choice nor power of precise prediction. There is a tragic dimension associated with the human condition which rightly makes us cautious about supposing that we can assess differentiated responsibility for life's misfortunates. And there are clearly many diseases in which lifestyle or personal choice plays no part, such as congenital anomalies.

In addition, objections can be raised about the simplistic notion of voluntariness involved in the merit argument. To argue that drinking, for example, is a purely voluntary act is to neglect the force of peer pressure, "social drinking," and advertising in our culture.

Finally, the merit argument evokes a scenario of old fashioned acts of "will power" as the solution to voluntary risks, thereby tending to "blame the victims" for their ill health.[25] As Dan Beauchamp says, "victim-blaming misdefines structural and collective problems of the entire society as individual problems, seeing these problems as caused by the behavioral failures or deficiencies of the victims."[26] Those who are convinced by the merit argument claim that our health care problems would be greatly reduced if only persons would refrain from disease-inducing practices. And this is, in part, true. But it does not follow that persons as isolated individuals, conceived as enjoying full voluntary control, are either the sole cause of their problems or the most effective avenue of remedy. The merit argument relies on a radically individualized sense of both health behavior and moral responsibility.

Some moral philosophers who readily accept a right to health care argue for a merit clause in the system of payments. Robert Veatch, for example, asserts that although persons who smoke, drink, and hang glide have an equal right to health care, they should be taxed for these voluntary risks to their health. Because they are more likely to use health care resources, such persons should be taxed at a rate calculated to add to the health budget an amount equal to the marginal health cost of their behavior.[27] Thus, Veatch's proposal would add responsibility for costs to the right to health care, retaining the basic right but modifying it along merit criteria.

The idea is attractive but not persuasive. In order to be a just system of merit, Veatch needs to show that not only do certain behaviors add to the expense of health care, but that the additional expense is greater than the costs of the alternatives. So that while a heavy smoker may die prematurely at age 50, incurring treatment costs for pulmonary diseases of $100,000, this may well be less than the alternative scenario of death at age 75, preceded by coronary artery by-pass surgery, multiple hospitalizations, and five years of care in a debilitated condition. It is not clear, simply from the economic viewpoint, that early death is a greater drain on resources. In fact, the reverse argument may be more cogent, that death is that great economizer, and that a just system—considered strictly on what costs we are likely to incur—should tax those whose health habits are likely to propel them into advanced old age.

Additionally, the notion of a merit-based tax system for health care would be contingent on an effective way to determine who was practicing what. While checks for seat belt usage seem easy enough, records of smoking, drinking, and other more personal behaviors would present significant practical problems. A true merit system would have to be accurate and reliable, and probably could not depend on voluntary self-reports. A health tax on cigarettes and alcohol at the time of purchase would be simple enough but arguably unfair unless other hazardous life-style habits were also taxed. An even-handed treatment for all such practices raises the specter of a health police, which violates cherished notions of privacy and liberty. It is unclear, beyond basic public health and safety criteria, that a merit system for personal health behavior could be made workable.

Mark Siegler invokes individual responsibility in a different way. In a thoughtful article entitled "A Physician's Perspective on a Right to Health Care,"[28] Siegler states that physicians have duties to serve the health needs of the public, but that the idea of a right is both ambiguous and deleterious. Siegler is chary of rights language for some of the same reasons discussed earlier in this chapter. Rights tend to be adversarial and turn quickly into absolute demands. Siegler claims this will undermine the doctor's freedom to do his job responsibly, restricting medical judgments and converting professionals into technicians. Medical consumers demanding specific treatments based on self-diagnosis will, Siegler claims, turn the traditional, covenantal physician-patient relationships into legalistic, contractual encounters. Siegler is, of course, correct, so long as rights are conceived in this individualistic and adversarial way. This is a basic misconception of rights and to the extent that the previous arguments are persuasive, Siegler's fears should be alleviated. In any case, Siegler's concerns, though legitimate, would have greater weight had he acknowledged that the reason why there is a fuss over rights to health care is because many are left out of the covenant. The current system provides no relationship at all, covenantal or contractual, for many in the greatest need of care. Contrary to Siegler, rights language is so fundamental to our moral and political heritage that we could not abandon it even if we wanted. A better alternative is the rehabilitation of rights to reflect a less individual and more realistic ethics.

The Right to Health Care and Human Needs

There is a moral right to health care, but not of the sort often claimed. It is a right grounded not in purchasing power, merit, or social worth, but in human need. The right to health care finds its rationale in a social concept of the self, in a sense of common humanity, and in a knowledge of common vulnerability to disease and death.

The right begins in a recognition that we all fall ill and are susceptible to disability and death. That is our nature and, whatever cultural variations there may be on this fact, the root awareness we have of this is not an invention but a discovery. Second, while some illnesses are self-induced, diseases generally are not the sort of things which are distributed by merit. We are all very likely to incur needs for health care for which we are not responsible and which are, in many instances, unforeseeable. Third, health care—largely as treatment by physicians, frequently as public health or preventive measures—is effective. Ill health is, in sum, the sort of thing which is universally experienced, but unevenly distributed, over which we have little control or predictive powers and for which there is frequently effective help. A just society is one in which the right to health care is based on the elemental fact of human need.

But to say there is a right to health care based on need is clearly insufficient. Everybody's needs are different, and it isn't clear whose definition of need (the physician's? the patient's? the Surgeon General's?) should be the standard. Also, in a consumer society we tend to express not only our true necessities but our hopes, wishes, and preferences as "needs." Occasionally we do this out of greediness and to legitimate our wants, but also because we sometimes lose sight of what our true needs are. Peter Singer, for example, argues that if everyone is granted health care according to need, there would be an obligation to buy everyone a car as well. Once need is recognized as a basic principle of distribution, Singer claims, there is no stopping short of a Marxist socialism.[29] This line of thinking hinges on a belief that all needs are alike and that health care needs are no different than a need for any number of useful commodities. Charles Fried presents a variation on this position in his argument for a "decent minimum" of health care for all, rather than equal access for all to whatever is available.[30] Fried doubts that people can genuinely benefit from many high-tech services, so it makes no sense to claim a right to them. But more importantly Fried, like Singer, thinks that health care is no different than many other needs people may claim to have. "Everything that can be said about health care is true of food and is at least by analogy true of education, housing, and legal assistance."[31]

Paul Camenisch provides a decisive rejoinder to both Singer and Fried. The "need" for a car is a socially created desire relating to status and appearances. While it may be inconvenient not to have a car, it is not on a par with not having working kidneys or not having effective medication. There is no satisfactory substitute for health care, and there is no way to live so as to make certain one will never need it.[32] Regarding Fried's more likely comparison of health care with food, Camenisch points out that the need for food is predictable and limited; "No one wakes up one morning needing $5,000 worth of food."[33] In another sense, food is more essential in that (unlike most medical care) there is a daily need for it. While food, shelter, and health care probably all belong on a "basic necessities" list, each is different from the others. If nothing else, our health insurance premiums should be convincing evidence that our health care needs are special because they are unpredictable and likely to be very expensive. Health care is sufficiently different from most goods and services so that establishing a right to it based on need does not propel us into Marxism or open the flood gates of insatiable demands for everything we might like to have.

It seems obvious that the concept of need will founder so long as it is individually defined and treated as a wholly private self-assessment. This assumption underlies the objections to need in Singer and Fried. Whatever needs are responded to with health care resources must be socially defined. This does not, of course, mean that a uniform set of needs should be imposed on everyone. Socially defined needs do not mean standardized or uniform needs. People differ dramatically in their actual requirements for medical help, and any list of needs which did not account for this would be unfair as well as foolish. Rather, needs must be socially defined in the sense that the recognition of what is basic and common among persons must inform the definition. One effort at such a basic definition is Norman Daniel's concept of health care needs as those things "important to maintaining normal species functioning."[34] Daniels believes that one can arrive at a principle of equitable distribution of health care resources based on species-specific needs as an extension of Rawlsian principles. Although Rawls may not provide a sufficient basis for recognizing commonality among people, Daniels' formulation of need is helpful here for it is fundamentally an appeal to a social perception. It implies human beings have normative, functional capacities which it is the proper object of health care to preserve and restore. That capacity is the condition for all particular goods which different individuals might like to achieve. No matter how diverse our vision of the good life, having an opportunity to realize it depends upon a rudimentary health to which we all aspire. The right to health care based on our need for it must appeal to this perception of a common good as the constant element in the achievement of diverse, individual life-plans.

To state it this way is to emphasize health care as an *instrumental* right. Health care is, of course, valuable for its own sake. Even when it is ineffective, we value being attended to and cared for by others. But health care is also valuable as a means to other things we deem important, such as autonomous functioning. Each of us can claim a right to that which is essential to equal opportunities, and it is primarily on this instrumental value of health care that our right to it hinges.

Others have also argued for an equitable health care allocation system. Amy Gutmann, for example, advocates a radical equal-access principle that would outlaw private markets for health care altogether.[35] This seems to me impractical and a position which places the wrong emphasis on the right idea. Gutmann seems more concerned about equality *per se* than meeting needs. In this way she seems to mirror her libertarian opponents who argue for liberty as an end in itself. But aside from a theoretical neatness, equality *per se* is no more a primary goal for health care than liberty. Equal access to health care is essential, but it is not the most basic goal. Equal access is important because now some have no health care at all. Equitable access is now the best means for meeting the goal of restoring persons to an equal opportunity to exercise their freedoms. An equal access in which all suffered more would not be a better system of rationing than an unequal system in which all benefited. This is, of course, the key idea behind Rawls' second principle.

A more complete statement of a right to health care is as follows: *A right to health care based on need means a right to equitable access based on need alone to all effective care society can reasonably afford.*

Equity based on need is to be distinguished from a sheer numerical equality. Health care resources should not be distributed according to a strict quantitative equality (one kidney machine for every family, or one psychiatrist for every one hundred people) since the need for care varies widely. In this sense, equality of services would not be equitable.

Equity based on *need alone* means that no one has a prior entitlement based on status, race, wealth, or other social differences. In the economy of health care needs, all similar needs are equal. Jones' needs are not more pressing or to be met before mine, just because he is Jones. Reagan may displace me for time and attention if he enters an emergency room when I am also a patient—there will always be extraordinary cases and exceptions—but generally, the existence of the need is *alone* the compelling factor for care, not the attributes of the person whose need it is.

The distributive principle of equity of care based on need contains within it a principle of restorative justice as well. The poor and disenfranchized, whose greater needs are related to previous, unjust policies of price-rationing, should get a proportionally larger share of available services. Restorative justice seeks to compensate for and repair past harms resulting from discriminatory practices. This is another way in which need-based equity differs from pure equality.

Effective care means that there is no obligation to provide useless or marginally useful treatments. Efficiency is a second criterion of justice, following equity and circumscribing its range. Effectiveness must be defined by those with expertise, largely physicians, nurses, and public health professionals. Effectiveness of care (and the resulting efficient use of services and facilities) is a necessary, but secondary principle. Where effectiveness and efficiency override equity of access, social judgments of worth come into play rapidly. Effective and efficient use of personnel and facilities must be established independent of who is being cared for. The selection committees who chose renal patients for access to scarce dialysis machines in the 1960s provide vivid testimony to the way in which judgments of effective use of resources easily gave way to judgments of social worth and merit. We must always ask "Efficient for whom?" Cost containment has become a shibboleth of health economists for the 1980s, as well it should, but there is a danger here of achieving efficiency at the cost of equity, and a neglect of the links between them. For example, a decline in prenatal care and immunizations leads to costlier (and less effective) care later on. It has always been more expensive to treat than to prevent most illnesses. Equity in essentials is not only more humane but cost effective.

What *society can reasonably afford* is a third qualification on the concept of need. A right to health care is not a license to demand care. It is not a right to the very best available, or even to all one may need. Some very pressing health needs may have to be neglected because meeting them would be unreasonable in the light of other health needs or social priorities. Health care is unique among needs and should enjoy a high place among our basic requirements for life. This does not mean that it should displace all else. My right to a kidney transplant, say, is circumscribed by a wide variety of factors which are ultimately decisions for society to make about the importance of this procedure: the number of qualified surgeons it trains, the network for histological matching it supports, the decision to have optional or assumptive kidney donor policies, and on and on. Tom Beauchamp and Ruth Faden put it well in saying that rights are inalienable (cannot be taken away) but not absolute. They can be validly overridden by more urgent claims or conditioned by social circumstances.[36] Rights are inalienable, yet contingent; contingent on the social matrix in which they are exercised.

How society will, through various political and professional means, arrive at decisions about what it can afford is an important question. The needs principle does restrict the responses and will eliminate any social ordering that does not recognize equity in meeting needs as fundamental. This means that while we may decide to allocate by disease categories, based on severity or prevalence, we could not justifiably distribute care by race or by money. The former are largely blind as to judgments between persons, and therefore express judgments that affirm the common vulnerability and need for health care. The latter are divisive, treating equal needs inequitably and judging the value of the need by a presupposed value of the person whose malady it is.

Finally, a right to health care is not a right to health. We cannot be entitled to something it is impossible to have, and no one can guarantee our health against the insults of living. Our over-medicalized culture tends to forget that. But a social right to need-based health care will have to remember its limitations in order to achieve what can be achieved with equity. To truly respond to needs we will have to return to a finite and intelligible set of expectations of what health professionals can do for us. In a purely negative sense, of course, we do have a right to health. Philip Lee and Albert Jonsen, for example, argue for a right to health that means, essentially, no one has a right to take away our existing health, or impair our functioning,[37] which would entail things like restraining polluters of air or water systems.

No health care system can alleviate all needs. As it stands, "wants" become needs, and needs which are met seem to create additional demands at a higher level of health. So some more realistic notion of needs will have to gain credence in our culture for needs to be a workable criterion. But this problem is not unique to the allocation principle favored here. Some curtailing of needs is required no matter what criteria are used for distribution.

Some—like the President's Commission—shy away from needs language altogether and prefer the notion of an "adequate level" of health care.[38] Yet it is impossible to define adequacy without recourse to a concept of need, and the President's Commission's report *Securing Access to Health Care* is itself a vivid testimony to this. To know what level of health care would be adequate we must know which health care needs it is important to meet. So 'adequacy' does not avoid 'need' but *presupposes* it. Frequently needs do tend to be thought of as bottomless pits, which would make satisfying them impossible. But the remedy for this is to strive for a workable and realistic notion of need, not to avoid it under euphemisms like 'adequacy'.

While all this argues generally for a social and more objective (rather than a wholly private and subjective) definition of health care needs, there is one arena where needs should remain individualized. At the level of first-contact accessibility, needs cannot be adjudicated by social or objective standards. To do so would turn patients into their own diagnosticians and eliminate one of the most basic services medicine provides. Primary care physicians separate real needs for care from conditions that do not

require or call for further professional intervention. Many
visits to physicians, perhaps a majority, are sponsored by
our ignorance or anxiety. Our need at this point is not a
need for treatment but a need for information and reassurance about our condition. And this need to know is so
powerful and pervasive—and so important to our personal
freedom—that it should not be subjected to rationing by
objective means. It is not clear how this could be done in
any case. But even if it could, it seems clear that in terms
of the need initially to be seen by a physician, each of us
is his or her own best judge.

Those who argue that need is not a good rationing criterion forget that in primary care this sorting out of multiple,
vague, and personalized notions of need is a large and
essential part of the primary care physician's role.[39] Many
of us are healthy hypochondriacs, and some visits to the
doctor are unnecessary, but the answer to this is health
education and less hype, not rationing which will inevitably
discriminate against some in genuine need.

Standard and less idiosyncratic criteria are required for
effective and efficient use of secondary and tertiary care
resources in order to curtail the frivolous and the fashion-
able. But the meeting of subjectively defined individual
needs at the primary care level is an essential and unavoidable part of the doctor's role. For the health care need
here is not necessarily for treatment, but for education,
information, reassurance, alleviation of anxiety, or just
human contact with an authoritative healer. To ration and
define away need at this level is to foreclose on equitable
access altogether.

Needs, socially defined, do not beg questions about
human nature, but do reflect a common experience in
which all eventually find themselves. All other criteria for
distribution reawaken individualistic modes of thinking,
for they depend for their force on what distinguishes and
separates us—wealth, talents, good looks, and merit, not to
mention guile and cunning in manipulating the system.

Principles of justice are intended to order social life. Principles too heavily dependent on individual norms or characteristics will obscure the common good which it is the object of justice to promote.

Rights language, which we so frequently use to make claims against society, can be used to express our desire *for* social cohesiveness. The principle of need in allocation of health resources is one such use. It signals the fact that health care is an expression of social solidarity. Rather than isolating us, the right to health care based on need reknits us into the social fabric where our needs may be identified through the sympathy of our fellows.

From Society to Community: The Needs of Strangers[40]

While many of the prominent theorists of justice begin with an image of the person as isolated and independent, we must recognize that our starting point is already one of relatedness. The perception of the self as social more accurately reflects our situation. It is to this perception that principles of justice must appeal.

Yet principles do not merely reflect perceptions. They sharpen and deepen them as well. The principles of equitable distribution based on need and restorative distribution based on past harms take us beyond a simple sense of social relatedness. To espouse these moral principles takes us beyond a sociality that is factual to one that is intentional. The social unity which these principles bespeak cannot be understood as primarily natural or biological, but as a unity self-consciously sustained by those who live within it. It is the unity of a community.

While we are all born into a variety of unchosen social arrangements and conditions, the notion of community emphasizes the chosen, moral expression of that sociality. While our social existence suggests a framework for a common moral life, it does not automatically provide it.

Indeed, ethical individualism of the sort we have discussed is a stance which denies any moral significance to social lineaments. But this individualism is itself a social expression —one that claims that all we have in common is a desire for non-interference and separateness. Such a minimalist ethics will finally undermine its own supports.[41] Neither individual rights nor social obligations make sense without the other.

Community, by contrast, seeks to affirm rather than repudiate the moral significance of social existence. Community recognizes and affirms what is common and expresses our sociality as a positive basis for action rather than as a confinement. The commonality recognized in principles of justice in health is the human condition of susceptibility to disease and death. The commitment to act in accordance with the principles of equity and need is a step toward reclaiming sociality as community. The will to respect vulnerability in all equally through equity of care is the foundation of community in terms of health care.

But a caveat is in order here. Concepts of community are too often nostalgic and utopian, evoking perfect harmony of sentiments and an organic solidity which submerges individual values. *Gemeinshaft,* as contrasted with *gesellshaft,* has frequently been used to denote the difference between 'community' and 'society.' Frequently *gesellshaft* (or society) stands for relationships built on rational calculations and mutual self-interests, such as are found in hospitals, schools, or courts, whereas *gemeinshaft* (or community) symbolizes relationships of deep bondage and nurturance, as found in families or small religious groups.[42] Appealing as it may sound, the organic notion of community implied in *gemeinshaft* is not helpful here. John Macmurray correctly claims that our wish for a society of organic and unproblematic solidarity is "a wish for the irresponsibility of the primitive."[43] Adherence to principles neither can nor should create a nurturing fellowship of intimates. We must still rely on churches, families, and friends, rather than social policy, for many of the important sustaining ingredients of selfhood.

In our larger national life we will always remain largely strangers to each other, and we will need a bureaucracy, with all the impersonalness it implies, to mediate whatever cohesiveness can be achieved by just policies of health care. Nonetheless, such cohesiveness can be substantial, and 'community' is not too grandiose an idea—when shorn of its utopian connotations—to express what is intended. A more realistic sense of community is one in which there are shared perceptions of the value of individual lives and a social commitment to protect them all equitably. Equitable recognition of needs is a prerequisite for community and equitable care for those needs is its goal.

The question of social justice in health care is: Are we willing to care for the needs of strangers? We have seen the power that identified lives have over us, and we all know of the deep pull to assist others who are close to us in blood, age, culture, and experience. These are all admirable and meritorious traits, what Smith would call examples of native sympathy, which is the wellspring of morality. Justice is the most arduous of virtues precisely because it requires that we extend these powerful motives to help to everyone and not confine them to those within an immediate range of concerns. Justice is difficult because it requires of us the impartiality which Smith espoused, as well as a retention of the sympathy which serves us so well in individual interactions. Sympathy directed by impartiality is a rudimentary definition of justice in health care.

So justice is difficult, but it is not beyond our capacities. We are aided in bridging the moral distance between recognizing our own needs and recognizing the needs of strangers by our basic sociality. But moral sentiments alone cannot guide morality; they only provide its source. Moral concern extended only to oneself is sheer egoism. Moral concern extended to identified and proximate others is virtuous, a primitive exercise of duty. Moral concern extended, in addition, to strangers directly encountered is benevolence or charity. And all of these are virtuous, in degrees. Justice is different because, more than any of these others, it requires imagination and intelligence.

The imagination required is the ability to imagine others who are not now present, spatially and/or temporally, as moral equals. It is this imagination which asks, for example, how much of our medical resources we should use so as not to leave the next generation with intolerable debts based on our desire for longevity.

We cannot identify all statistical lives, thereby giving them distinctive names, faces, and histories. The nation is too large and too diverse. Moreover, as Jonathan Glover pointed out, the effort to identify and sympathize with all persons and their plight would probably be purchased at the cost of psychic health. The idea of identification and extension of sympathy to *everyone* is a regression to the romantic notion of an all-inclusive and intimate community. It is counterproductive as an ethical proposal because it is impractical. It enjoins an impossible ideal, and is thus irresponsible. So while not all lives can be identified, all lives are *identifiable*. The moral imagination at work in sympathy makes us cognizant of our situation and the limits of our ability to feel the needs of others. Though we may never know directly the needs of strangers, we can know that those needs exist. An impartial sympathy, a sympathy disciplined to see its own provinciality and thereby deepened and extended in principle to all persons in society, bridges the gap between identified and statistical lives. Need-based equity expresses the insight that strangers are identifiable and that their health care concerns are as powerful to them as ours are to us.

Intelligence is called for because justice requires ethical reasoning at a higher level than for individual morality. Instinct, custom, habit, and good will can carry us through a great number of one-to-one encounters quite well. Justice, by contrast, requires adjudications of principle at many turns and a kind of thinking which calculates probabilities and weighs consequences for large numbers of people.

But prior to each of these requirements of imagination and intelligence is the insight that we are not immune from the suffering of others even if they are strangers. To the extent that we isolate ourselves and count anyone's suffering as insignificant, to that extent is our own humanity diminished. It is this insight that sympathy suggests, and principles of equity spell out. A health care system which neglects the poor and disenfranchized impoverishes the social order of which we are constituted. In a real (and not just hortatory) sense, a health care system is no better than the least well-served of its members.

5. The Physician's Role and Policies of Rationing

We in the U.S. are currently rationing access to health care primarily by price, and secondarily by disease, by race, and by age. This rationing scheme has for a long time remained unacknowledged as such because it fits so snugly with capitalistic values and a consumer mentality. Such an approach relies on the virtue of charity to deal with those who are excluded from access to care. While such benevolent gestures were never adequate, the combination of recent hard economic times, uncontrolled health care costs, technological innovation, and egalitarian social sentiments have made it evident just how far this scheme deviates from a just system of allocation.

Lester Thurow claims that in health care we are both capitalists and egalitarians. We believe in the free market mechanisms that allow the rich (and the insured) to buy whatever health care they want, yet we also are unable to let the poor (and the uninsured) suffer or die because they cannot afford an available treatment.[1] The result is the mishmash of *ad hoc* rationing that depends on media appeal and personal pleas for marginally effective high-tech procedures. When successful, these appeals and pleas bankrupt local social services budgets for routinely effective treatment for a great number of the poor.

In viewing the moral ingredients which lie behind this approach we have seen that a way out of this problem is a renewed sense of community, grounded in an awareness of our social character as human beings and our innate affinity for social life. A need-based equity in the allocation of health care resources is the measure of a just system. Even so, "needs" must be defined and to some extent curtailed, for no health care system can serve all the needs, even all the legitimate needs, a population may have. Who shall make such adjudications? Who should ration health care? It is part of the genius of the market system of rationing that we are protected from asking this moral question by the aegis of individualism and the inflated notions of liberty and independence which go with it. A devotion to this *form* of rationing lets us off the hook from asking the *substantive* question of whether the outcomes of this system are just. The virtues of liberty and self-reliance are thought to be so closely tied to this form of delivering services that suggestions about alternatives are frequently unthinkable or are conceived exclusively as abridgements of freedom. It is clear that liberty is better preserved in a more equitable system of health care, but still we must answer the troublesome question of who will ration services. Even in the best of worlds—where selfish, personal, and vested professional interests are kept at bay, where a sense of community and social responsibility prevails, and where needs are adjudicated rationally and equitably—the actual rationing must fall to someone. Who should do it? At what level should it occur?

The Physician as Rationing Agent

Lester Thurow contends that doctors should do at least a major part of the rationing. He suggests that if third-party payers write rules and regulations concerning what they will and will not pay for (and prohibit going outside the system) the machinery will be stiff and work clumsily. "No set of rules can be adjusted to the nuances of individual medical problems."[2] Thurow's plan would have physicians making decisions which dissuade patients from treatments or procedures which are not justified by the marginal benefits. This would require, of course, reliable information on the effectiveness of alternative treatments and a serious effort at technological assessment prior to dissemination. Thurow adds that the norms for "bad medicine" should be expanded "to include cases in which high costs are not justified by minor expected benefits."[3]

The virtues of Thurow's system would be flexibility and preservation of judgment at the point closest to the actual rendering of care. Thurow implies, but does not state, that physicians are likely to make better judgments about what is expendable and what is not in health care. And he, like most observers, believes that controls on cost are inevitable; if physicians refuse to make these choices, those less capable eventually will.

Physicians, by contrast, have almost uniformly objected to assuming the role of rationing agent. The argument seems to be an ethical rather than a technical one. Most physicians seem to object to others allocating resources, implying that they themselves are best qualified to do it; but at the same time, physicians eschew the rationing role on moral grounds. Sometimes this is combined with a denial that rationing is needed; Marcia Angell, for example, argues that it is "premature."[4] Norman Levinsky presents a recent example of this reticence in his response to Thurow. Physicians, he says, "are required to do everything that they believe may benefit each patient without regard to costs or other societal considerations."[5] Howard Hiatt states a similar conviction: "A physician or other provider must do all that is permitted on behalf of his patient."[6]

The scenario that Levinsky, Hiatt, and others have in mind is not, however, the prudent withholding of marginally effective and expensive treatments which Thurow suggests, but the sacrifice of a patient for a social agenda of conserving resources. Levinsky, to be sure, is not a vitalist who argues for a maximalist philosophy of life at all costs. He is concerned that once a social agenda of conservation is raised, the doctor will be in the impossible position of serving two competing masters, the patient's good on the one hand vs. the social good on the other. Here the tug is between the deontological duty to benefit a particular patient and the utilitarian calculus of "the greatest good for the greatest number." Levinsky sees the problem, then, as one of divided loyalties and one which is impossible of resolution except in favor of the individual patient. Citing the errors of probability estimates, bias against particular groups such as the aged, and differences in experience and expertise, Levinsky claims that there are practical as well as moral reasons for not putting rationing decisions in the physician's hands. Society, he says, not doctors, must decide how to limit the availability of medical services.

Levinsky's position has much to commend it. Trust and the assumption of beneficence toward each patient are key ingredients in doctor-patient relationships. These might well be compromised if the physician assumes a role as rationing agent.

Yet Thurow and Levinsky may not be as far apart as it at first appears. They seem to be responding, at least in part, to differing scenarios. Thurow's recommendation is for more prudence in the use of expensive treatment at the margins, while Levinsky is properly chary of a crass (or even a subtle) attitude of expendability of individuals for a social good. Levinsky's position suggests a mental slippery slope in the physician's morality, such that once a social good becomes visible at all, it will threaten and perhaps overcome entirely the physician's traditional duties to patients. Benevolence to individual patients is here taken as an absolute norm which will abide no admixture and rises or falls as a sole and sovereign principle. When the evidence for benefit is ambiguous or soft, Levinsky seems to fear that even the presence of a social agenda will mislead physicians and skew their intentions and motives, creating new occasions for disregarding a patient's well-being.

Despite these clarifications, the core disagreement remains. Thurow believes physicians should decide when patients are to forego treatment at the margins; Levinsky believes the margins are usually ambiguous and that adding a second agenda of social good invites abuse. Thurow says that doctors are in the best position to ration; Levinsky says they must not ration for morally significant reasons.

The limitations on both points of view should be mentioned. Thurow has not had to do the rationing he recommends and has never felt personally the tug of conscience of which Levinsky speaks. Levinsky, though clearly well-read and thoughtful, is limited by the patients he sees and with whom he identifies. He cannot, in the very nature of things, be as appreciative of the needs which are denied when the policies he advocates are followed. It could be argued that the limitations of both men are such that neither has a viable grasp on the problems. Each has an important point which should be preserved and incorporated into a larger perspective. The three points which follow are offered in order to push the inquiry further and clarify some of the misconceptions on both sides.

1. The first and perhaps most important item to notice is that we are already rationing care as a society, and that physicians as a profession are already rationing care. As a group, physicians have lobbied intensively for the current structure of health care. Thus at the larger socio-political level, it can fairly be claimed that physicians have never been free of the burdens many of them do not wish to have. It will be objected here that complicity in the larger system of price allocation is not the same as rationing care on a case-by-case basis. Roger Evans, for example, makes a major distinction between *allocation,* as macrolevel policy decisions, and *rationing,* as microlevel decisions about distribution to individuals.[7] This is a helpful distinction for clarifying the various levels on which decisions are required,

but it can not be used to suggest that we are not currently rationing, or to isolate physicians from responsibility for the kind of system in which they work.

It is too easy to say that physicians are not rationing because they don't decide between patients or withhold care to preserve the public purse. To draw a line around one's actions with the selected group of patients one happens to see personally is to succumb to precisely the sort of individualistic morality that has sustained the inequities in health care for so long. Physicians are responsible, as all of us are, not only for the quality of care they give to the patients they see but also for the characteristics of the access system within which they work. Physicians are not, of course, totally responsible for the larger socioeconomic structures of medical practice. These structures are sustained by a variety of sophisticated cultural and economic forces to which we all contribute. But because physicians have claimed for themselves professional prerogatives over how they shall practice, they have an added degree of responsibility for the macrorationing which marks our current system. Moral persons and moral practices cannot be completely separated from the larger context in which they work. The same is true, of course, for all professions.

This is not to impugn the motives or intentions of individual physicians nor to suggest that the moral traditions which guide physician conduct are wrong. However, these traditions are inadequate, lacking as they do any social reference or sense of public accountability. The problem is not malevolent professions as some, such as Illich, would have us believe. Rather the difficulty lies with honorable professionals doing good in a sphere artificially bounded by a socio-political philosophy and undergirded by a moral tradition which systematically excludes reference to the larger society. Taking off these blinders will be disturbing, for the larger picture is one of inequities and neglected needs.

Reinhold Niebuhr remarks that William Lloyd Garrison

attacked both slavery as an institution and slaveholders. By contrast, Mohandas Gandhi could separate the imperialism of English policies in India from individual Englishmen whose virtues he could respect.[8] Even the latter example may imply too much for many readers, but it underlines the point forcefully. Good done within a circumscribed sphere of action must always be weighed against a clear-eyed veiw of the larger cost of that good. Even the most virtuous of physicians cannot claim immunity from the larger context of forces which limits the healing which they achieve. Many of those who are most aware of this are, of course, physicians themselves, and I owe my best insights into this dichotomous ethics of responsibility to my physician colleagues.

2. Acknowledging a degree of responsibility for the current system of rationing health care does not mean that a physician's primary duty is to protect the public purse. Withholding needed beneficial care from one patient in order to benefit others violates a variety of norms, both general and medical. The physician's primary obligation is still to his or her patient. But this does not preclude a secondary obligation to use resources wisely and to desist from marginal and very expensive care. The care of the individual patient is a powerful norm, and it is the first obligation of doctors, but it is not their only obligation. Conserving resources cannot exist side-by-side as an equal with individual loyalties, but this does not mean that the obligation to conserve scarce and needed resources is not real.

None of us have the luxury of loyalty to only one principle or the simplicity of unambiguous devotion to one and only one person or set of persons. Most of us hold a variety of roles which are potentially conflicting and must be sorted out. We may have emotional and financial obligations to a spouse, children, aging parents, extended family, and others. While some ties take priority, the other obligations do not cease to exist. Physicians who are members of university faculties have duties to their institutions, students, and house officers as well as their patients. Sometimes these duties conflict and a careful sorting out is required, but such a task is not impossible. In a like manner it is not pernicious to suggest that physicians have a duty to conserve resources, and that this is largely compatible with, though secondary to, a primary allegiance to individual patient well-being. I as a patient would not be suspicious of a physician who articulated his or her loyalties in this way. Indeed, I would be far more dubious of someone who claimed that he or she never considered cost or the possible waste of resources in considering my treatment. Unalloyed allegiance is an impossible standard of purity of motive, and anyone who believes themselves capable of it may be subject to other overestimates of their virtue and ability as well.

To say that physicians are, and to some extent must and should be, rationing agents does not mean they should be making policy on the spot. The American Medical Association, as early as 1959, recognized the need to ration, but unfortunately saw it as an individual and *ad hoc* endeavor to be exercised only with poor patients. The House of Delegates declared: "The individual physician and the medical profession as a group must also be concerned with maintaining a proper balance between adequate medical care for the welfare patient and economical use of public funds."[9] Clearly this is unsatisfactory. Guidelines and policies developed at a higher organizational level are necessary, and this is possible without the straitjacket of regulations which concerns Thurow. It is the denial that rationing policies are needed at all which engenders the *ad hoc* responses which we now have.

3. Frequently the claim that moral factors prohibit physicians from rationing is combined with a claim that "patients want no less."[10] Here the idea is that physician-patient relationships will be jeopardized by concerns for cost and conservation. Patients expect and demand total

allegiance, untainted by social concerns. This sounds honorable but even prior to cost consciousness and equity concerns, some social obligations are present. Some infectious
diseases require reports to protect the public, as do certain
other medical conditions for persons in jobs of responsibility, such as bus drivers, soldiers, or candidates for
public office. So there is already precedent for protecting
the commons that, while not uncontested, is largely
accepted. A medical commons depleted of resources
because of physicians who are zealous for all treatments
possible and/or a public clamoring for longevity constitutes
no less a hazard to our well-being in the long run.

Moreover, there are groups in society who would not
have their life extended at the margins at great expense. [11]
Christian doctrines of stewardship prohibit the extension
of one's own life at a great cost to the neighbor. This is not
fatalism but a simple matter of proportion. Most patients
would not bankrupt their family and deny their children a
fair start in life by striving for a last, expensive extension
of their own lives. An imaginative sympathy shows that
neither should we extend our lives at the margins if by so
doing we deprive nameless and faceless others a decent
provision of care. And such a gesture should not appear to
us as a sacrifice, but as the ordinary virtue entailed by a
just, social conscience.

Underlying attitudes of stewardship and proportion is
the conviction that life is not an unblemished good nor
death an unmitigated evil. Older traditions (Jews, Christians,
Stoics, Moslems) have always believed it was important to
die at the right time and for the right reasons. This is not,
of course, to romanticize death, or to suggest that it is not
sometimes tragic. The death of children is always so. But
we cannot pursue longevity with such a passion as we now
manifest and at the same time remain faithful to the spirit
and meaning of our lives in community.

If the next generation is to flower and flourish we must
practice the wisdom of giving ground when our time comes.

This will be distressing only to those who think they are entitled to indefinite extensions. Leon Kass has put it definitively in claiming that our expensive efforts at longevity at the margins are, in any case, a situation of not knowing our own needs. "Man longs not so much for deathlessness as for wholeness, wisdom, and goodness." [12] If Kass is right, then we should not object to a social factor in our care, but in fact require that physicians not strive too long and at too great an expense to preserve us. Justice requires that our individual needs be the physician's first obligation. But justice also requires the imagination and intelligence to recognize that there are limits to all loyalties. Our right to receive care is itself a socially established right and, as such it cannot help but be responsive in its claims to the social context from which it draws its meaning.

British Rationing and American Rationing

The British National Health Service (NHS) is probably the most widely studied foreign health care system, and comparisons with the U.S. have been frequent. As there are many studies available, there is no need to repeat generally understood facts about the NHS here. It is worthwhile, however, to focus on some of the cultural differences that make the NHS a viable system for the British, one in which most Britons have considerable pride, and, more specifically, on some of the ways British physicians act as rationing agents. It would be foolish to suggest that we can or should simply emulate the British, but perhaps the peculiarities of our traditions and practices will become more clear as we look at another way of doing things.

Rudolf Klein, one of the sharpest observers of the NHS, sums up some of the major cultural differences.

> Britain is an original sin society in which illness and debility are seen as part of the natural order of things

and patients tend to be deferential. America is a perfect-ability of man society in which illness and debility are seen as challenges to action and patients tend to be demanding consumers.[13]

These cultural differences in expectations of health and of medicine's relative power to cure go a long way toward an understanding of why the NHS, and the rationing it entails, are supported in Britain.

The NHS provides universal health services to everyone at little or no cost to the patient at the time of rendering care. This includes almost everything from ambulatory visits to sophisticated surgical procedures entailing lengthy hospitalization. Health care is conceived explicitly as a basic right of citizens, and it is the role of government to provide it. The underlying objective, as described in the legislation creating the NHS in 1948, is "to secure . . . that there would eventually be equal opportunity to access to health care for people at equal risk."[14] Thus the NHS is a system of centrally planned and funded distribution of health resources following roughly a principle of need-based equity. Need is further refined by reference to criteria such as the population of a given area, its age/sex ratios, and morbidity (measured as standardized mortality ratios). Additional factors such as overlapping service areas, educational needs, and capital investments for facilities are also weighted in the current allocation formula.[15]

Such a system does not provide everything for everyone (no system can), and in many cases there are severe limits on what is available. While access to a general practitioner (GP) is readily available to all in Britain, there are long waiting lists for many surgical procedures. For hip replacements, for example, it is not uncommon for patients to wait two years or more. There are as well a variety of both formal and informal understandings among both patients and doctors about who will and will not receive treatments that are expensive and scarce. The elderly, for example, are ordinarily not dialyzed for chronic renal failure. Generally, infants under 700 grams are not aggressively treated. These are but some of the instances, both implicit and explicit, of rationing policies. Obviously such rationing is required. Budgets are set every year at the highest government level, and districts and health institutions within districts are required to stay within these limits.

So one way in which the British control the demand for care in a nationalized system is by controlling the supply. If very few intensive care units, dialysis machines, or tissue matching programs are available, individual patients are less likely to claim that they are discriminated against when they do not have access to therapies which require these resources. Since no money ordinarily changes hands, there is little inclination to think that more money will buy better care. Also, there is a small, private medical care market for the few citizens who do want to buy out. This provides a safety valve for wealthy and vocal dissatisfied citizens who might otherwise skew or overload the NHS by their demands.

Among the factors that influence the allocation of hospital resources in Britain, Henry Aaron and William Schwartz list the following:

(1) *age* — for example, lack of routine access of the elderly to chronic dialysis;
(2) *fear of the disease* — radiotherapy for cancer is readily available;
(3) *visibility* — hemophilia, which is visible, is more widely treated than angina pectoris, which is not;
(4) *aggregate costs* — hemophilia treatment is expensive but there are only a few new cases each year;
(5) *capital funds cost* — CT scanners are scarce because of large acquisition and maintenance costs;
(6) *costs of alternatives* — hip replacements are done because the alternative care of a disabled patient is higher than the cost of the procedure.[16]

Of special interest is how British physicians function as rationing agents, saying the "No" to patients that Thurow believes must enter the vocabulary of American physicians as well. Aaron and Schwartz describe the process as one of a constant search for rationalizations. Whenever possible, they contend, British doctors look for medical reasons to carry out their gatekeeper role. The denial of a treatment is made to seem routine or even optimal, so that nothing of real medical significance is lost in not referring a patient to a treatment center. For example, an elderly person with failing kidneys may be told that no really effective treatments are available, or that such treatments would be painful or extremely burdensome, and that the patient would be better off without it.[17]

This may sound like gross discrimination and deception to many Americans accustomed to unquestioned access to all that can be done. It is hardly surprising that British doctors would need to frame allocation policies in terms of medical factors. To tell any person that they are being denied care because of scarce resources is always difficult, and there is always the wish to avoid implications that those who are not treated are less valued as individuals than those who are treated. Yet it is not the value of the elderly as persons that is in question but the relative effectiveness of chronic renal dialysis in relation to other medical and social needs of the citizenry. Such a policy decision, while not easy or simple, has nothing of the moral opprobrium of a decision, say, to dialyze citizens of London but deny equal resources to residents of Brighton.

Moreover, there is some indication that British GPs do not self-consciously ration as often as one might think. In some cases, outmoded standards of practice may prohibit GPs from referring patients to consulting physicians at regional treatment centers. Sometimes ignorance of novel procedures may act as a rationing force, so that no conscious decision to deny or dissuade a patient from seeking further treatment is called for.[18] This is, however, far from desirable, even if it relieves physicians of a burden. In other cases, patients themselves may not expect or desire further treatment. An innate sense of egalitarianism pervades the NHS, the sense that resources are genuinely limited and should be shared out as far as possible across the whole population. There is no doubt that lower expectations for expensive treatment combine with an egalitarian spirit to diminish the requests for additional treatments. Finally, there are the traditions of deference to physicians and diminishingly few malpractice suits which assist in the overall acceptance of rationing by both patients and physicians.

So there is no doubt that rationing occurs in Britain and that British physicians, especially GPs, are key figures in translating these policies to their patients. Rather than a mercenary denial of patient rights, however, it seems to be generally perceived as a necessary correlate to a system which strives for equity with limited resources.

Americans who are appalled at the more explicit rationing policies of the British should remember that the U.S. is not free of such actions, but speaks of them in a guise which leaves the rationing factors implicit and *ad hoc*. The British have decided that access to a GP should not be conditioned by money, but that access to expensive high technology must be controlled by the factors discussed above. Americans, by contrast, have decided to restrict access to primary care by price, but have given universal, free access to some groups when they became impossible to ignore, even when the treatments are only marginally effective. One system is planned and controlled rationing, the other is rationing by default, with scatter-shot advocacy forces at play to adjust or by-pass the market. One system inevitably requires its practitioners to be agents of rationing, the other largely claims that rationing violates medical standards of ethics. The burden of these observations has been to indicate that American physicians already do ration care, and further, that it is inevitable and proper that they should assume some responsibilities in this process. British

GPs do not make policy in the clinic, and they are supported in their decisions by a cultural tradition more realistic than ours about perfectability and longevity. Whether we can support American physicians as they are called on to help make and enact these hard policy choices will be a major test of our cohesiveness and even our viability as a society. Whatever future policies are enacted must not continue the present practice which combines an official denial of the need for rationing with *ad hoc* policy decisions at the bedside.

Policies of Rationing and Distribution

Principles of ethics, even those universally accepted, do not lead with simplicity to policies. Many adjudications and interpretations are needed to translate moral convictions into action. Principles of justice in health care are no exception. Yet to leave off policy considerations altogether would imply an abstractness and irrelevance to ethical reflection. Ethics rarely tells us exactly what to do, but it can and must give some sense of orientation and direction.

Primary and Basic Health Care

Equitable access based on need to all effective health care which society can afford will mean, first, an accessible system of primary care physicians and other providers. Citizens must have an entrance into the health care system. If this does not exist, care ceases to be both equitable and effective. An accessible system of primary care is necessary not only to meet the immediate needs of the ill but to implement successfully the proper use of more sophisticated and expensive resources. The Institute of Medicine definition of primary care offered in 1978 is an admirable statement and fits the requirements of justice well. The Institute's study report on "A Manpower Policy for Primary

Health Care" defined it as "accessible, comprehensive, coordinated, and continual care provided by accountable providers of health services."[19] Such providers are in the best position to give the sort of basic or minimal care that is foundational. Included in basic care should be immunizations, basic health education, inexpensive curative therapies (e.g., antibiotics for bacterial infections), inexpensive therapies which give symptomatic or temporary relief for chronic conditions (e.g., insulin for diabetes), emergency care, palliative care for incurable illnesses, care for the elderly, the mentally ill, the physically and mentally handicapped, and hospitalization as needed to achieve these ends.

Accessibility will require considerations of geographic distribution and whatever requirements are called for to establish this network of coverage. Maldistribution might be resolved by more effective incentives to locate in rural or inner-city areas, or by uniform requirements to practice for a limited time in underserved regions. Obligatory requirements of limited duration do not seem disproportionate to the investment society makes in its medical practitioners.

Universally accessible primary care meets several needs: first-contact and coordination of future care; personal security to individual patients; and symbolic affirmations of equality within a commons. Each of these are important, and the first two are perhaps obvious. The symbolic dimension deserves elaboration. Primary health care available to all without restrictions of cost, location, or other factors will create a sense of solidarity and community. It relieves the need for competitive individualism in which my health needs can be met only if someone else's are not. It affirms that in vulnerability to illness, all are equal, and no further legitimation or enfranchisement is required.

At the primary care level a relatively pure equity must reign. To begin to adjudicate needs before or in the absence of this sort of basic access is to ask patients to diagnose themselves and to discriminate against those who cannot. At this most basic level, physicians should not be saddled with the burden of protecting the commons, or in any way ration care between individuals. What rationing must be done at the primary care level should be done by policies set at a higher level, which govern availability of additional resources.

Some have argued that instead of a direct provision for health care services, the poor should be given cash. Milton Friedman prefers this method because he believes direct services are paternalistic, while cash would allow the poor to buy whatever services they choose, including none at all, if that is their preference.[20]

There are several problems with Friedman's proposal. The goal of a health care system is not to augment consumer liberty, *per se,* but to meet health care needs. The poor are usually not only lacking in money, but are restrained in other ways that may make their use of health monies less than prudent. A choice between health insurance and food or clothing, for example, is hardly a free market decision. Moreover, giving money is not morally the same as giving services, just as buying and selling blood is vastly different from receiving and giving it on a voluntary basis out of a community's altruism.

An accessible system of primary care will in some instances also satisfy our concerns about efficiency and costs. Prenatal care, for example, can be extraordinarily cost-effective. Most observers believe that every dollar expended on care before birth saves between two and eleven dollars on mothers and infants after birth. Similar savings are likely to accrue from early treatment of many chronic conditions, such as hypertension and diabetes.

Our current system rations at the point of initial access, which is frequently the least expensive and most effective point of encounter between doctors and patients. Ironically, we seem to ration expensive, high-tech medicine far less frequently. A recent example of this irony can be found in the report of the Federal Task Force on Organ Transplantation. The Task Force recommends that public and private programs extend their coverage of heart, liver and other "extrarenal" transplants to all citizens who need them.[21] If this recommendation is enacted, no doubt many of the indigent previously excluded would receive new organs. And yet—setting aside questions of whether these transplants are proven therapies—the result is a policy of honoring equity in extreme cases while ignoring it in basic care. It perpetuates a system which values identified over statistical lives, heroics over effectiveness, cure over prevention, and a rescue ethics for a few over basic care for many.

Additional Health Services

At a higher level of decision-making, the policy makers must employ norms of utility as well as equity. Utility considerations for our purposes here can be stated briefly as "the greatest good for the greatest number." Policy making at this level should take account of factors such as the relative effectiveness of therapies, prevalence and severity of diseases, and the overall health needs of society. So limits will likely have to be put on the sorts of treatments offered, based on their overall effectiveness and the social importance of treating one sort of malady rather than another. For example, decisions may have to be made as to whether it is better to build burn centers or expand neonatal intensive care units, whether to focus on arthritis or diabetes in research protocols, or whether to transplant hearts or mount intensive coronary prevention programs.

Equity is still a key criterion, however, *within* each program that is undertaken. For example, if utility dictates that additional beds are to be added to the intensive care unit, all who need them must have equitable access to those beds. Jones, though he might buy his way out of the queue altogether, cannot buy his way ahead of Smith within the queue and preempt Smith's right to equitable treatment. While the primary and basic care level offers a more complete equity, at the macrolevel utility is the overriding consideration in making policy. Equity in administering the policies is essential, however.

In addition, equity may come into play in a second way. Suppose that a group of persons suffer from a disease resulting from an inequity of risk that has been socially encouraged or tolerated, such as diseases peculiar to coal miners, asbestos workers, or those who handle vinyl chloride. Here fairness requires greater expenditures to assist those persons under the principle of restorative justice. Their relatively greater needs are the result, in part, of social practices and priorities from which many benefit. Therefore, attention to their work-engendered diseases should override ordinary rules of utility.

At no point should physicians be asked to choose between or among individuals and try to assess who is to be included and excluded from care. A well-known and important example of the trauma of such efforts to choose is the experience of the Admissions and Policies Committee of the Seattle Artificial Kidney Center at Swedish Hospital. Early in the 1960s when renal dialysis was in its infancy and dialysis units were scarce, this Committee was given responsibility to decide which patients among the large number suffering from End-State Renal Disease in the Seattle area would be granted access to the small number of dialysis machines. After certification of "medical acceptability," the criteria adopted by the Committee included age, gender, marital status, number of dependents, net worth, educational background, occupation, past performance, and future potential. At one time the Committee even solicited and received letters of recommendation from neighbors and employers in order to assist in their evaluation of candidates. The application of such criteria proved exceedingly problematic. The problems created by this and similar processes of selection helped lead to the universal availability of dialysis in 1972, in a revision of Medicare legislation. Universal access at no cost to the patient eased the dilemmas of doctors and selection committees, but it created even greater problems at the policy level. Estimated to cost no more than $50 million at its peak, renal dialysis now costs taxpayers almost $2 billion per annum, for 75,000 patients. While these patients are only .25 percent of the Medicare B population, they use over 9 percent of the Medicare B resources—funds which might have been used for other medical needs.

Whether this allocation of funds is disproportionate is a question to be decided in relation to other uses and their relative importance. The point is that choices between identified individuals is an impossible task. The requirements of utility are different in that selection is made among diseases or categories of diseases, on the basis of malleability, frequency of occurrence, morbidity, expense of treatment, and so on. For example, it is not absurd or hopelessly biased to decide, on the basis of available intervention, that some forms of cancer should not be the purview of curative medicine, but of only palliative care. To decide that resources should go into prevention is not to abandon or discriminate against some cancer patients; it is simply to attempt a rational assessment of effective intervention. To fail to attempt such an assessment would be unjust overall.

The general order of priorities for treating these needs should be a social choice, though more particular decisions will need to be made by experts and professionals. For example, it should be a social choice as to whether a network of primary care providers is made available to all citizens, but those with greater expertise would need to decide just what is to be included in such a package. As it now stands, intense political lobbying accompanies many decisions about whose health care needs are funded. In addition, the power of professional specialty groups in medicine to command resources is considerable, especially when energies are focused on a well-publicized case or a particularly dreaded illness. All these factors are relevant, but none should hold hegemony over allocation choices. A well-formed social choice will not be swayed excessively by consideration of the peculiar maladies of prominent families or the odd assortment of diseases which interest incumbent U.S. Presidents; a more rational, less emotional process is called for than sponsoring a disease of the month or calling for a "war on cancer." Careful information and expert advice is needed but should not be decisive in such a social process, and the need for much public discussion and a general consensus is clear.

One such ranking of needs follows. In this scheme, resources would be devoted to (2) only after (1) has been fulfilled, and (3) only after (2), as funds permitted.

(1) very expensive therapies which sometimes effect a partial cure or temporary remission (e.g., chronic renal dialysis, some treatments for hemophilia);

(2) very expensive therapies of ambiguous benefit; (e.g., liver transplants, perhaps heart transplants);

(3) elective procedures that satisfy personal desires or correct minimal burdens (treatments for baldness, cosmetic surgery).[22]

Whatever ordering of health priorities is devised at the policy level, it must have a component for technological assessment. Currently technologies are devised, marketed, and rapidly disseminated in ways that prohibit adequate assessment of their relative value. Without either a theory or methods of proper assessment it is likely that new technologies will appear and evolve in ways that make their value difficult to discern and their allocation inefficient and unjust. No serious effort at allocation can succeed without a robust program of technological assessment.

In summary, this general outline strives for equal access to all for primary and basic health care. At the primary care level, individuals must be free to discern when the attention of a professional is called for. Primary care providers should decide if basic care is needed, and if so, equity of access at this juncture must reign. Here physicians must decide, in collaborative relationship with patients, what kind and how much health care is needed. Use of resources appropriate to need and proportionate to expected benefits is the goal. Both physicians and patients should be aware that some very expensive therapies may be precluded by policies established at a higher level. The physician would retain flexibility in judging what primary and basic care is needed, but some options for additional care (especially costly and marginally effective care) would simply not be available. This would not lead to an adversarial doctor-patient relationship, for the doctor can still advocate for the patient and provide all that is within available limits. Physicians must not be held responsible, morally or legally, for not trying every conceivable last-ditch therapy if they are constrained by prudent and just policies. Such a system might also allow for a reduction of the cumbersome and ineffective review mechanisms.

At the level of additional care, some services would likely be available while others would not. Utility in the use of limited funds would be a key criterion at this larger policy level. Equity would continue to be important in two ways: within available programs, discrimination against individuals would be disallowed; and some priority would be given to those whose maladies are the result of past social injustices.

Such a system would, of course, be far from perfect, but it would be more just than the current one and a system in which citizens could have confidence. Justice depends on a rationing system that is as explicit as possible, where the rules are fairly arrived at and administered, and where rationing practices are not out of accord with sound medical judgments or well-informed social choices.

Preventive Medicine vs. Rescue Medicine

It is easy to argue for the benefits of prevention but difficult to enact policies that favor prevention over rescue. Preventive services are defined as those measures which we can reasonably expect will help to avoid or lessen the prevalence or severity of an illness. Rescue services are responses to present and identified health problems in particular people. There are at least three dimensions of this set of choices that are morally interesting.

The first dimension is the different responses we have to identified vs. statistical lives. The problems in responding to statistical persons with illnesses would remain, along with some additional factors. Preventive medicine seeks to alleviate problems that not only are just statistically real, but are not now existing. Thus the second facet of these choices is one between present versus future problems. Prevention addresses problems that may arise in persons *yet-to-be* identified, which puts it yet one more step removed from the rescue impulse. Moreover, the payoff from preventive practices usually cannot be measured for some time to come. Treatment of essential hypertension is a good example here. Hypertension is frequently asymptomatic, and even to understand the threat it poses, a person must project probabilities (not certainties) of avoiding premature death (not tomorrow but in twenty or thirty years). It is no wonder that compliance is at best sporadic and largely confined to those who perceive the future as something to which they look forward. Perhaps this also explains why the health community likes to couch their educational programs to hypertensives as "treatment" rather than prevention. Hypertension exemplifies those odd twilight zone maladies that exist in the present but whose sickness-making characteristics all lie in the future.

Third, and more from the perspective of those rendering services, there is a difference between value-rational and goal-rational considerations.[23] Value-rational behavior focuses upon the symbolics of the action, what the action expresses about the agent and the recipient of care. Goal-rational behavior is more logical and concerned with outcomes, consequences, or goals. Thus, while providing rescue is always value-rational because it expresses concern for the sick or injured, policies which overwhelmingly favor rescue over prevention may not be goal-rational and justifiable in terms of efficacy and overall usefulness. Some transplant surgeons, for example, frequently invoke the symbolics of rescue and discourage questions about the extent to which their actions are warranted on other grounds. Prevention services are usually thought of as goal-rational since those who are affected are not yet known and would require rescue only in some future time.

How to adjudicate the relative merits of prevention vs. rescue is not soluble here. Good data will perhaps ease some of the tension by indicating just which preventive services are truly effective and, also, which rescue services are only symbolic. It is easy to forget, in the zeal of rescue, that many interventions involve imperfect technologies and exact a price in suffering as well as resources. It is unclear how many purely symbolic gestures of rescue we can afford. The burden of these arguments has been to show that we are putting our symbolic gestures of care in the wrong place. A very expensive gesture to one person which has little hope of lasting success should not be seen as a replacement for providing effective, inexpensive care for others. Gestures of heroism have too often overshadowed gestures of justice. Commitments to equity in prevention and treatment are also powerful symbols and can be seen as value-rational as well as goal-rational.

Some will suggest that there is something wrong with persons who are not moved to do all that is possible for present victims of illness, in favor of future needs. Perhaps this is true, but it is not a greater flaw than ineffective rescue efforts of those presently before us which jeopardize present or future persons. Unless we are content to give in altogether to the rescue impulse, we will eventually have to admit that there are hard choices here. But to admit that there is tension, that choices are likely to be difficult and often tragic, is no more or less than to acknowledge that we are human and moral, and not gods.

The Purpose of A Health Care System

Paul Starr has said that "if one wishes to equalize health, equalizing medical care is probably not the most effective strategy."[24] But equalizing health is surely not the goal of a health care system. Whatever merit there might otherwise be in it, equalizing health is an impossibility. Health depends on a variety of factors, of which medical care is but one. Some critics have questioned whether even health, never mind equality of health, is a goal of the current health care system. If health care is bought and sold on the market it does leave us open to charges like those of Michael Michaelson, that "health is no more a priority of the American health industry than safe, cheap, efficient, pollution-free transportation is a priority of the American automobile industry."[25]

Talk of equality in health, beyond basic public health measures, is unrealistic and values egalitarian ideals over effective action. The purpose of any health care system must be to meet health care needs and to do so in as just a way as possible. This will *not* result in equal health, but it should result in equitable access to health care resources. The hazards of assuming that equitable access will lead to equal health is well illustrated in the debates in Britain over the past five years.

Britain is a country committed to an equitable system of health care based on needs, yet in 1980, a study on inequities in health indicated that the differences in health status among social classes in Britain remain untouched by the effort to share health resources equitably.[26] Although the health of all Britains was improved, the difference between the health of Social Class I (professionals) and Social Class V (unskilled laborers) was as great as it ever had been.

These results should not be surprising. Differences in health status result from differences along many axes, not just access to care. Nutrition, housing, health education, life-style, socioeconomic stress, and the general ability to use the system of services are all factors in health, and all relate to class differences. This indicates that equitable access can help but not overcome or compensate for other factors in health status. So the relative gaps among and between the classes cannot be eliminated by attention to health services alone. It may also be that it takes several generations for equitable access to resources to show up in a more equitable health profile.

Another way to express the point at issue here is through the difference between input and outcome. Pure equality in outcomes, while desirable, is utopian. Attention to outcomes are important, lest resources be wasted, but attention to outcome alone, with expectations of equal health for all, overlooks essential forces at play in health and makes us forgetful of some essentials in health care itself. In seeking care we value the process as well as the outcome, and indeed the process is sometimes all there is.

To value equality *per se* is the opposite mistake to valuing efficiency *per se*. The recent history of legislation from the U.S. Federal Government provides a case in point, for here the emphasis has been on controlling costs, not enhancing access or improving quality. Certificate of Need legislation (CON) for example, beginning in 1974, has focused on preventing excess capacity in state and local planning regions. Vague goals and lack of real sanctions have hampered the effectiveness of such planning. But the point is that even if CON legislation had been effective there is no reason to believe that access to health care would have been more equitable. There are no measures to ensure that the more limited supply of facilities would serve the underserved and there is no plan to use the potential savings from these cost-control measures on better services for the underserved.

Neither equality nor efficiency by themselves are worthy goals of a health care system. Both mistake means for ends. The goal of health care is, quite simply, to meet needs. To do so without reference to equality in access or efficiency in outcomes would be unjust. But this does not mean that equality or efficiency are goals worthy of esteem by themselves as measures of health care. A health care system should be one means of assuring equity of opportunity among citizens, but equal health will no more result from it than equal intelligence will result from high quality, equitable public education.

Getting clear about the purpose of a health care system should make us cautious about enthusiasm for many cost containment measures, for some of them seem likely to achieve cost control at the expense of the most vulnerable. The Diagnosis Related Group (DRG) Prospective Payment scheme of Medicare adopted by Congress in March 1983 is the most recent example of measures which deserve close scrutiny.

Under the DRG system hospitals are reimbursed not according to costs incurred but according to the nature of the patient's illness. Upon discharge, each patient's stay is placed into one of 471 categories depending upon the principle diagnosis, secondary diagnoses, complications of the hospital stay, age, sex, and other factors. The hospital reimbursement is then calculated according to this formula. If the hospital stay costs less than the reimbursement, the hospital keeps the difference. If the care is more expensive, the hospital must make up the difference. The incentives are just the reverse of previous payment schemes, for here more efficient health care is rewarded.

The implications of DRGs are far-reaching. Danielle Dolenc and Charles Daugherty call it nothing short of a "counterrevolution" in health care financing.[27] Many believe these or similar measures of cost control will be adopted by many state governments and private insurance carriers as well.

It is easy to see why DRGs are so attractive. Medicare accounts for 40 percent of all hospital revenues in the U.S., and some believe that if the present growth rate of costs continue, Medicare will soon face enormous deficits.[28] DRGs put the stress at the point of major decision-making —the doctor. Physicians control roughly 60 to 80 percent of all hospital costs through decisions about admissions, tests, length of stay, and ancillary services.[29]

The tension this places on the physician is obvious, although obligations of efficiency have always been present.[30] Our concern is less about reduced quality for individual patients than about reduced access to the underserved. Instances of discharging patients prematurely or neglecting needed procedures will be minimized by the reluctance of physicians to deny care to present, identified patients with whom they have formed relationships. The greater danger may be in a tendency to reduce accessibility to the sicker-than-average or the lower-than-average DRG reimbursements. Since the solvency of the hospital will depend on the attraction of a favorable DRG case mix, attracting DRG-favorable patients and discouraging DRG-costly patients could become the newest form of rationing. A rationing such as this is very likely to harm the poor, since their lower health status makes them generally more costly to treat. Proprietary hospitals, run by multinational corporations, will have even less incentive to think of an entire community's needs and not to skim the most favorable patients while systematically discouraging the rest.

The prospective payment scheme of Medicare is only one of the recent strategies being promoted to increase efficiency. Health Maintenance Organizations seek efficiency by serving only a defined population with capitation financing, while Preferred Provider Organizations rely on price discounting and utilization controls. These strategies are designed to increase competition (and thus efficiency) among physicians and among provider organizations. Yet competitive systems have winners and losers, and this sort of terminology may in itself diminish any sense of collective responsibility in health care.

Prior to the competitive emphasis, hospitals were able to care for some non-paying patients by charging paying patients more. The new methods of reimbursement make this very difficult. In a competitive market for health care, the subsidization of the poor will be diminished or eliminated as groups with favorable ratings demand insurance rates that truly reflect their low utilization. As Victor Fuchs says, "The current trend is for each group to get the lowest possible premium for itself, regardless of what happens to the rest of the community."[31] Hospitals which provide care at lower and more competitive rates can ill afford the philanthropy of the past. There is already evidence that this is adversely affecting the poor, especially poor children.[32]

While there is nothing *prima facie* wrong with physicians being advocates of efficiency, there may well be irreconcilable gulfs between the goals of profit and equity. Careful study will be required to determine if prospective payments, "experience" rather than "community" ratings, capitation, and utilization controls alter the goals of health care and thus subvert the requirements of justice.

A final clarification is needed to prevent misinterpretations. Our chief concern here is the just distribution of health care resources, not primarily questions of how health care is financed or how physicians and other health professionals are paid. It is clear that the fragmented, market-driven system we now have leaves much to be desired. It does not follow from this that markets should be outlawed altogether in health care, which would in any case be impossible. Nor should anyone read into the emphasis on sociality a simplistic endorsement of "socialized medicine"

—a hortatory phrase (or scare slogan) without precise meaning.

There are a wide variety of ways to organize and finance health care. None is, in itself, morally good or evil. Each should be judged by the yardstick of need-based equity, rather than for its fit with a political or economic ideology. There are likely many paths to the goal of a more just system. The question is whether we are *willing* to take them.

Conclusion: Reconciling Samaritanism and Justice

In California Koren Crosland received a liver transplant paid for out of state funds by order of the Governor. In Illinois Amy Hardin's family and friends raised $265,000 from private resources to pay for her liver transplant.[1] In Florida, Billy Bostick received half a million dollars through the largesse of a Saudi Arabian prince to pay for a new heart and lungs.[2] Other children whom we cannot name suffer from similar problems and die, away from our attention.

We in the U.S. currently live in and support a health care system which provides inadequate or no care for 20 percent of our population. The rest of us receive a graded level of excellence based on our ability to pay. The uninsured, if they survive at all, become the recipients of an *ad hoc* philanthropy, rescued by the heroism of virtuous individuals. Such heroism is surely admirable, but reliance on heroism is a bizarre way to run a health care system. There aren't enough Saudi princes to save all the Billy Bosticks, or even to assist those whose chances of survival are better.

We can no longer turn away from the recognition that a market-driven health care system is a *de facto* rationing scheme. Our scatter-shot policies have produced a system of reactive programs designed to patch and plug a price-rationing system. The result is a secondary system that rations by age (Medicare), by disease (End-Stage Renal Disease), by media appeal (parents pleading for livers), and by provider philanthropy. We keep the acknowledgment of rationing in the background through the use of optimistic (sometimes utopian) assessments of our abilities and our needs. The hard choices of scarcity, we tell ourselves, can be avoided by efficiency, technological innovation, cutting the defense budget, or outproducing our needs. In fact, no society has been able to avoid rationing its health care services. The only question is how to do it justly.

For Americans, however, this will not be easy either to recognize or to achieve. The genius of the American self-image—individualism, self-reliance, progress, and prosperity—predisposes us to an ethical individualism and makes us forgetful of our interdependence and social connectedness. Our health care attitudes bespeak a norm of sovereign solitude on the part of both patients and providers.

The models of justice we most frequently work with are of no help with this problem. Rather than enhance our ability to think socially, these models cripple it and blunt the perception of our rootage in a social world antecedent to our private and personal lives. The system of Rawls, no less than Nozick or Engelhardt, views the just society as a self-conscious construction fabricated from individual self-interest. Not only does it pretend to a sovereignty of choice we do not enjoy, it fails to give any significance to the social web in which even our most personal choices reside. Justice cannot be properly conceived as a simple extension of an individualistic view of man. A just health care system, whatever its final shape, requires a recognition of our sociality and mutual vulnerability to disease and death.

Individual self-sufficiency, which was a virtue in the American frontier of the past, has become a vice in our late twentieth-century thinking about health care. A more mature ethics will not discard self-reliance but temper it with social concerns. What is needed is not just an alternative but a larger context. Individualism in health care is debilitating when taken as our highest or only value, but in a social context it can be a valuable propensity.

It is a flawed moral philosophy that must pit the dimensions of our moral sensibilities against each other as irreconcilable antagonists, as if we must be either individual or social, private or public, solitary or communal, rational or affective, self-interested or altruistic. The truth about us is more complicated and frequently ambiguous, for neither side of these dualities is even comprehensible in isolation from its complement. The supposed opposition between ethical individualism and sociality is finally false. The moral life is irreducibly social, as well as inexhaustibly individual. The opposite of sociality is not a rugged and isolated individualism but moral anarchy.

Working our way out of the current modes of rationing care and into a more equitable system will require an examination of our values which we have heretofore been loath to make. While difficult, such an examination is not beyond our ken. Resources for social responsibility are dormant but not absent. Awakening our awareness of social links and ending the hegemony of possessive individualism in health care does not threaten our identity as distinct individuals. Nor does social ethics thwart our liberty. For the moral understanding entailed in atomistic anthropology is severely depleted and cannot finally command our respect. Flat-footed assertions of the moral life as freedom, merely and *per se*, without reference to the right conditions of its exercise or the social dimensions of its meaning, are romantic idols. The social sensibilities outlined here, such as sympathy, compassion, and justice, do not provide a full picture of the moral life, but they do move us in the right direction. Finally, it is not just specific virtues or values such as freedom that are at stake in how health care is distributed. At stake, as well, is the coherence of life, lived out over time and in community.

Liberal and libertarian traditions of ethical individualism have ushered in a season of medical ethics in which justice is depleted of any social significance. They seek to pluck the fruit of freedom but see no obligation to nurture the communal vine from which it flowers. Rawls, Nozick, and Engelhardt are only the most prominent of those who think that it is possible to understand justice as the extension of individual moral character, conceived as private, solitary, and free. The burden of this essay has been to indicate the flaws of these efforts and to point to other traditions which can serve us in developing a just health care policy.

Traditions of civic virtue and social responsibility are not missing in America, just dormant. A full explication of these traditions is not attempted here.[3] But at a minimum, remembering these traditions would lead to a "recovery of a sense of civic life as a form of personal self-development."[4] It is essential that American society explore and reaffirm the qualities of life that go beyond a possessive and solitary fixation on self.

A just health care system is not the only expression of renewed social sentiments, but it is a very important feature of our common concerns. Striving for justice when people are most vulnerable is one way of translating latent social concerns into a common language.

A better understanding of ourselves as social creatures leads to a reconciliation of Samaritanism with the claims of justice. Ethical individualism leads us to believe that these two moral requirements are inevitably conflicting. A better grasp of our situation does not automatically preclude all conflicts between these ideals, but puts each ideal in the context of the other.

It is not Samaritanism *per se* that is faulty, but the individualism we bring to that parable that leads us astray. Properly understood, the story of the Good Samaritan is not an example of philanthropy or largesse, but of the impetus to help that springs from common vulnerability and recognition of need. The biblical term is 'compassion', to suffer with; the term of eighteenth-century Scottish philosophy is 'sympathy', an imaginative sharing of another person's condition. Both indicate a primordial, human, responsive capacity that takes us beyond the isolated and self-interested rational calculators which inhabit modern theories of justice. The anthropology of Locke, Rawls, and Nozick makes justice an artificial and contrived virtue. Beginning from a more adequate view of the person shows that the basis of justice is already within us in the form of social passions and social interests that constitute us as individual selves. Thus we do not have to create or fabricate our social life from a calculating self-interest but can follow at least some of our uncalculated social instincts to begin to build a just society.

Samaritanism is best understood as a sign of our social nature rather than a supererogatory overcoming of alienated and egoistic motives to condescend to help another. Justice is Samaritanism enlivened by an impartial imagination. An impartial imagination is one which has learned to recognize its own biases and the tendencies to assist only the identified others of our experience. Principles of justice deepen and extend this innate sympathy, naming the social context of our motives and extending the range of our actions to those beyond our immediate life. Justice is Samaritanism chastened by awareness of its parochialness and enlivened to the larger world.

Case Studies

Case Study 1:
Rationing in Life-Threatening Situations

Consider the following incident adapted from a report by Jerry Bishop in the *Wall Street Journal,* December 10, 1981 (p. 33):

> A young woman was rushed to an emergency room with internal bleeding.
>
> After 25 days the patient left the hospital alive and well. The cost: $358,942.88, of which the patient's out-of-pocket cost was $17.50 (for telephone calls). This may be the largest bill ever run up by a patient for a single illness episode.
>
> Factor VIII inhibition, the woman's ailment, is unusual; fewer than 50 cases like hers are found in the medical literature (and the drug to combat it accounted for $333,858 of the woman's bill).
>
> The methods by which the bill was paid are going to raise hospital bills for thousands of other patients and their health-insurance carriers. The patient was covered only by Medicaid, and the total reimbursement for her care was limited in this case to a total of $12,600.

Questions:

- Was the right decision made in this case?
- Are there alternatives?

- Should cost have been considered?
- Who should decide these questions?

Commentary:

Let us consider this case from multiple perspectives: the physician in charge, the blood bank director, the director of the hospital pharmacy, the hospital's general directors, and from the perspective of state or national planning.

The physician in charge of this woman's care should not be the rationing agent. Efforts to conserve for society, made at the bedside, are bound to involve the physician as a double agent. Indeed the actual physician in charge in this case said, "We knew we were getting into big money, but we had no choice." The decision to let an identified patient die in order to assist unknown others may be a price no psyche can bear. If we as a society are to retain the trust of physicians, we should not expect them routinely to ration at the bedside or perform in other ways that violate their sense of integrity.

Let us change the case slightly. If this patient also had an underlying terminal and irreversible illness, treatment for her factor VIII problems might have been considered useless or futile. In this situation, a decision not to treat vigorously but to offer only palliative care might be made on sound medical grounds. If the patient and family concur, no question of a breach of fidelity could be raised. The physician is simply following prudent and ethical practices.

To say the physician in charge should not be a rationing agent here does not mean that he or she is obligated to do everything possible. It would be imprudent to empty the blood bank or to use all the very expensive hemophilia medication on this one patient, thereby denying resources to other patients, including those with classic hemophilia. But the point is that it is unfair to give the physician in charge free reign over this matter. It is unfair because it presents a situation of unavoidable conflict and because it isolates the decision and the physician as decision-maker unnecessarily. The decision should not be this physician's alone. The directors of the hospital blood bank and the hospital pharmacy should be helpful here in establishing policies within which physicians can work.

The blood bank director's responsibility is not to one patient or another as individuals, but to all patients in the hospital. If a single patient uses resources which deny adequate or safe care for many others, the blood bank becomes ineffective and forfeits its larger mission. Deciding how much is too much for any given case is always a relative judgment, and no exact rules are likely to be applicable. Yet a policy of review of the demands for blood products along roughly utilitarian lines would preserve the integrity of the blood supply. It would also relieve the physician in charge of sole responsibility for decisions of when enormous expenditures become too burdensome because other patients are jeopardized.

At an earlier point, policies in a hospital pharmacy should also serve as a boundary condition for the range of the physician's actions. The initial decision to place the hemophilia drug in the hospital's formulary is a resource allocation choice. Some hospitals, for example, small community hospitals, may choose not to stock a remedy for factor VIII inhibition because they simply cannot afford it. Other hospitals which on past experience know that a small number of hemophilia patients with this particular problem are likely to seek care at their institution may decide to purchase a small quantity to handle emergencies that arise. It is one thing to stock $40,000 worth of anti-inhibitor coagulation complex for emergency use. It is quite another to skew the hospital's supply budget by keeping on hand all that may conceivably be needed, costing perhaps several million dollars.

At yet another decision point, the hospital directors may decide that certain very expensive procedures or products simply will not be available at their institution.

For example, several years ago, prior to the advent of cyclosporins, some hospitals decided against offering heart transplants. High costs and questionable benefits combined to deter Massachusetts General Hospital in 1980, and this decision was not rescinded until 1984. Thoughtful and sound choices at this level may also relieve physicians of *ad hoc* decisions and preserve the autonomy of patients, families, and doctors to decide for themselves in all but a few restricted cases. Hospitals, like pharmacies and blood banks, must sometimes protect themselves (and their usefulness to patients overall) by prohibiting overzealous physicians or patients through policies which extend services to as many as possible. To refuse to consider such policies guarantees unfairness and results in an inefficient and irresponsible use of resources.

Finally, from the perspective of state or national planning, policies must be made which will use resources wisely and will not pretend that all things are possible. But the problem is not just making such policies. Following prudent policies has proved to be even more difficult than making them. In the past few years, we have seen increases in dramatic and heart-felt pleas from parents when policies denied coverage to their children. For a governor, congressman, or other public official to refuse the burden of rescue would likely be political suicide. In our zeal for saving lives in this way, we usually forget all the good reasons for the policies which disallow access or payment for some very expensive and marginally effective therapies. And when the therapies fail we console ourselves with the thought that "everything was done." This is a heavy price to pay to alleviate our guilt. Other patients, as yet unidentified, also pay a price in terms of services not received. Such patients, disproportionately the poor and minorities, cannot command the attention of their elected leaders to the same degree as an attractive, terminally ill child and a set of articulate and determined parents. The death of such a child is tragic, but the depletion of a complete health care budget for a long-shot therapy is even more so.

Decisions about the fair distribution of medical resources require analysis at many levels. Adopting appropriate policies at each of them will enhance good decision-making with patients and families, preserving a great deal of autonomy at the point closest to care while circumscribing the scope of available choices in a prudent way. Patients and families will be less tempted to try to circumvent policies they understand and believe to be reasonable and equitably applied.

Case Study 2:
Rationing in Ambulatory Care

It is 8:30 P.M. in the general medicine ambulatory clinic in a large hospital. The patient is a 46-year-old married white male with long-standing hypertension controlled by thiazides. He enters the clinic with complaints of chest pain of approximately 12 hours duration; the pain was present on awakening that morning. It is a severe substernal pain that he finds hard to describe—it isn't exactly a burning, but rather a "deep ache." It isn't really crushing or pressure-like, but neither is it sharp. The pain has waxed and waned in intensity, but never gone away completely. The patient has stayed at home all day (it is Sunday) and has engaged in very little physical activity. He does think the pain increased when he walked out to the street to get the paper and was made worse when he drank hot coffee.

He admits to "several beers" the night before. There has been no nausea, vomiting, or hematemesis. Baking soda and Alka-Seltzer gave transient, partial relief. Overall, the pain seems a little better, but the patient thought he better have it checked out before bedtime.

The family history is significant for the death of his father at age 52 with acute myocardial infarction. The patient currently works as a heavy equipment operator. The initial physical exam is normal.

Questions:

- Are rationing considerations involved in the care of this patient?
- What values or priorities are implied by the ambulatory care setting? By the time of day? By the patient's presenting illness?

Commentary:

The physician is here faced with rationing of at least five different resources.

The first is time. Even if no other patients enter the clinic, the physician chooses between this patient, reading a medical journal, going home to family, or other worthwhile activities. Rationing time involves decisions about how complete a history and physical exam to take, how far to probe in the family patterns, social supports, or potential conflicts this patient may have at home or at work. Spending more time gathering this information now may save time later on, but there is no assurance of this. Moreover, patient expectations of appropriate physician behavior can figure into the choice of how much time to devote to these items. Even if it seems clear, on purely biological grounds, how much of a history to take, the social and cultural context of this encounter may also play a major role in influencing this allocation choice.

Time is related to the second resource which must be allocated, namely reassurance. If the physician's role is to comfort and relieve suffering as well as cure, reassurance must also be considered as a resource to be distributed along lines of prudence and proportion. Too much reassurance may give the wrong impression, in this case that everything if fine. Indeed, it may be very hard to tell if all is fine and honestly offer the "clean bill of health" we have mistakenly come to take as a guarantee of long life and vitality. Verbal placebos, or other gestures of reassurance and symbols of care are sometimes expanded to include sugar pills or dummy medications, complete with prescription pads and prices. Here questions of truth-telling get mixed into the picture. Reassurance can be rationed according to need (the patient's or the doctor's), according to the physician's feelings about frankness and honesty, or titrated to suit particular patients in particular circumstances. Hypochondriacs, the "worried well," will always want more of it than most physicians are inclined to dispense. A patient who presents himself at the clinic at 8:30 P.M. with chest pain and has a family history of heart attack is clearly in search of reassurance. How much he receives is a product of many factors.

Rationing reassurance may also involve a third resource, namely diagnostic tests. Laboratory tests, x-rays, and a variety of other studies may, like words and prescriptions, be used as placebos. The temptation to do so may be especially strong if a patient has been to another physician and not received a satisfactory explanation. Patients sometimes come to a large hospital or academic center to get all that medicine has to offer, the latest techniques from the best and the brightest. Using diagnostic tests for their placebo value alone is usually not sound practice. Not only does it risk a false reassurance, it also reinforces patient expectations which are already inflated and unrealistic. In addition there are the costs of the tests to consider. Even if the patient does not directly pay for such tests, someone eventually will. Diagnostic tests not based on biological indications tend to be ineffective and inefficient overall. Some patients who have too high a regard for the specificity or sensitivity of tests may have their expectations altered by counseling and education, but this implies a judgment to use more of the first resource discussed, the physician's time.

When there is a genuine question about the usefulness of a test, the problem is more complex. There may be pressures from colleagues to use or not use certain procedures that serve institutional or departmental needs. Some tests are labor intensive and to get them may involve calling in additional personnel, long waiting periods, or a return visit. Other tests may be encouraged by the very presence of a piece of technological wizardry, or by the need to pay for or justify expensive equipment through frequent use.

Other factors which may be involved in rationing tests are fear of malpractice suits, fear of being wrong and responsible for an unnecessary death, a maximalist philosophy of care, the education or appearance of the patient, the patient's degree of anxiety or desire for the test, monetary gains or constraints, and on and on. In the best of worlds these factors only influence rationing at the margins, but as we know this is not always the case. The physician who orders tests for purely biological reasons alone is rare, and even so, it is not clear that acting solely on biological indications is the best medicine.

A fourth scarce resource this physician must ration is access to a specialist. Should this patient be seen by a cardiologist, or even by another general practitioner for a second opinion? Patients may, of course, call for appointments and be seen by specialists on their own, but being referred by another physician is a smoother and more authoritative path. Many of the same considerations which influence the use of tests also affect decisions about referral to specialists.

A fifth rationing decision concerns the use of hospital beds. Should this patient be admitted? Again, the same pressures are likely to apply, along with some additional ones. If the hospital is part of a Health Maintenance Organization, there is economic incentive not to use a hospital bed for ambiguous or marginal cases. By contrast, if a hospital has a falling occupancy rate, the pressure may run in favor of hospitalization. Whether this patient has insurance may be a factor in how much of any of these services he receives.

A primary care physician should never be involved in choosing between patients in life-threatening situations. Moreover, physicians at this initial level of care should be free to determine, in collaboration with their patients, how much care is appropriate. Good quality care for the patient is the physician's first norm, with the larger needs of society and the virtues of efficiency and conservation playing a secondary role. Getting clear about this is important, but even so, it does not resolve all the problems. As this case illustrates, the possibilities for rationing care are almost limitless, and this will be so as long as physicians maintain control over the operations of the health care system. Some may see the rationing role as an unwelcome burden or the result of a misguided ethics. This case illustrates that rationing has been and continues to be a necessary and unrelinquishable task of physicians. Like all tasks, it can be performed skillfully or clumsily, but when placed within larger standards of good care, it need not be inimical to the traditional loyalties of physicians to their patients.

Case Study 3:
Rationing in Decisions about Health Care Programs:
An Exercise

The Federal Government has placed a cap on any new health care expenditures. The eight programs listed below have been proposed for funding. The total cost of all programs would be $30 billion, but only $17 billion is available. Which programs would you select for funding? Rank them in order of priority, and distribute the available funds.

A. Continuation of the Renal Dialysis Program
   ($2 billion annually for 75,000 persons).
B. Institution of a Comprehensive Prenatal Health
   Program
   ($2 billion annually. Black infant mortality rates
   are double those of white).
C. Expansion of Neonatal Intensive Care Technology
   ($1.5 billion annually for 200,000 infants).
D. A Totally Implantable Artificial Heart Program
   ($3 billion annually for 25,000 people, when per-
   fected).
E. Health Insurance for the Uninsured (*employed
   and unemployed* and their family dependents
   who are not covered by private insurance, Medicare, or any other insurance program)
   ($8 billion annually for 25 million persons).
F. Expansion of Cancer Research
   (by $2 billion annually).
G. Improve Health Care Coverage for the Elderly
   ($10 billion annually for 27 million persons.
   Many elderly require long-term care in skilled
   nursing facilities. They are admitted as private-pay
   patients and "spend down" to Medicaid eligibility
   only after their assets are depleted).
H. Continuation of Support for Persons in Persistent
   Vegetative States (e.g., Karen Quinlan), with artificial feeding and hydration, antibiotics, etc.
   ($1.5 billion annually for 10,000 persons).

Question:

- What ethical principles support your allocation of
  the $17 billion available?

Commentary:

   The programs listed above are all legitimate contenders
for funding. The figures given for each are approximate,

but not unrealistic. Many other programs could be added or substituted for some listed here. The overall assumption of a ceiling on expenditures for health services is daily more evident.

There are many ways to choose which programs to fund. The list below is a sample, together with a justification for each choice. There is no single right set of choices, but discussion of what and why we choose as we do should move the discussion beyond the purely intuitive or emotional level and allow for debate on the merits of each program.

1. *Pure egalitarianism* would refuse to consider the particular merits, efficiency, or needs of the recipients of each program and simply divide all the available monies equally. Each program gets equal shares (and most are underfunded), at $2.1 billion.

2. *Equitable egalitarianism* would give each program an equal percentage of its request, roughly 50 percent. Unlike pure equality, here needs and numbers come into play after considerations of equality.

3. Assist the *neediest* first, or the *most ill* first. This policy would seek to rescue those nearest to death. In this scheme renal dialysis and neonatal intensive care units and persons in persistent vegetative states would get their full requests first, likely followed by the artificial heart program.

4. Seek *the greatest good for the greatest number.* Here 'good' must be defined, but at least one way to determine this is to ask which programs will effectively help the largest number of persons. This mode of reasoning would likely place health insurance for the uninsured at the top of the list, followed by improved health care for the elderly.

5. Choose in accordance with *long-range efficiency and effectiveness.* In this mode of reasoning, priority will be given to prenatal programs, which are quite effective in avoiding many neonatal problems,

and cancer research. Both programs appeal to a preventive emphasis and eschew expensive and frequently ineffective rescue efforts.

6. Act on the principle of *restorative justice*. Choosing this principle, greatest assistance would be given to those whose maladies are caused or exacerbated by previous social or economic injustices. If this logic is followed, prenatal programs (which affect many minorities) and insurance for the unemployed (losers in a competitive economy) would be given top priority. Cancer research might also be a favorite under this system of allocation, since some forms of cancer seem to be prevalent in lower socioeconomic groups and may be the result of an environment more foul for the poor than for other citizens.

7. *Honor long-standing obligations.* Here a moral criterion for ranking programs is loyalty to those who have previously been treated or to whom one owes fidelity due to past obligations. Following this criterion would place renal dialysis patients and the elderly at the top of the list. Both groups, it could be argued, deservedly expect our care because of our past relations with them.

8. *Draw the winners from a hat.* This is the lottery approach, used as a measure when all programs are thought to be equally meritorious or when the relative worth of the programs affected cannot be (or should not be) judged. Proponents of a lottery say it gives everyone an equal chance. Opponents claim it is like "throwing dice" and is a choice "by default."

Notes

INTRODUCTION

1. Howard H. Hiatt, "Protecting the Medical Commons: Who is Responsible?" *New England Journal of Medicine* 293 (July 31, 1975): 235-241.

1. THE REALITY AND NECESSITY OF RATIONING

1. The phrase, as well as this contrast, was taken from Thomas H. Murray's "Ethics and Health Care Allocation," *Public Law Forum* 4, no. 1 (1984): 41.

2. Thomas A. Preston, "The Artificial Heart and the Public Purse," *Medical World News,* September 10, 1984: 94.

3. See Doug Lefton, "Public Hospital Limits Care to Tampa's Poor," *American Medical News,* April 20, 1984, and also the *American Medical Association News,* February 1983.

4. Ronald Bayer, "Getting to the Heart of Things," guest editorial, *The New Physician,* April 1985: 7.

5. H. Arnett Ross, III, David R. Kusick, Sally T. Sonnefield, and Carol S. Cowell, "Projections of Health Care Spending to 1990," *Health Care Financing Review* 7, no. 3 (1986): 3.

6. Roger W. Evans, "Health Care Technology and the Inevitability of Resource Allocation and Rationing Decisions," *Journal of the American Medical Association* 249, no. 15:2047-2053.

7. Ibid.

8. Ibid.

9. Robert M. Gibson, Daniel R. Waldo, and Katherine R. Levit, "National Health Expenditures, 1982," *Health Care Financing Review* 5, no. 1 (Fall 1983): 9.

10. Lewis Thomas, *The Lives of a Cell* (New York: Viking Press, 1974), 31–36.

11. For a useful discussion of this problem and its implications, see Alain Enthoven's *Health Plan* (Reading, Mass.: Addison-Wesley, 1980), 16ff.

12. The best critique of the vitalistic perspective is Joseph Fletcher's *Morals and Medicine* (Boston: Beacon Press, 1960), 172–210.

13. Aaron Wildavsky, "Doing Better and Feeling Worse: The Political Pathology of Health Policy," in *Doing Better and Feeling Worse,* ed. John H. Knowles (New York: W. W. Norton, 1977), 108.

14. Ivan Illich, *Medical Nemesis: The Expropriation of Health* (New York: Pantheon Books, 1976), 76–77.

15. Karen Davis and Diane Rowland, "Uninsured and Underserved: Inequities in Health Care in the United States," *Milbank Memorial Fund Quarterly* 61, no. 2 (1983): 149–152.

16. Ibid.

17. President's Commission for the Study of Ethical Problems in Medicine and Biomedical and Behavioral Research, *Securing Access to Health Care,* vol. 1, (Washington, D.C.: U.S. Government Printing Office, 1983), 55. Although infant mortality rates have declined overall over the past few decades, the discrepancy between black and white rates has increased. See U.S. Department of Health, Education, and Welfare, *Health, United States, 1979* (Washington, D.C.: U.S. Government Printing Office, 1979), 11.

18. Davis and Rowland, "Uninsured and Underserved," 157. See also M. E. Levin and L. S. Levin, "Health Care for the Uninsured," *Business and Health* 1, no. 9 (September 1984): 9.

19. Ibid., 163, 165.

20. U.S. Department of Health, Education, and Welfare, *Lead Agency Memorandum on a National Health Insurance Program* (Washington, D.C.: U.S. Government Printing Office, April 3, 1978), 6, as cited in *In Search of Equity,* ed. Ronald Bayer, Arthur Caplan, and Norman Daniels (New York: Plenum Press, 1983), xiv. See also the important study by John Kosa, Aaron Antonovsky, and Irving Zola, *Poverty and Health: A Sociological Analysis* (Cambridge, Mass.: Harvard University Press, 1969).

21. President's Commission, *Securing Access* 81–82.

22. Ibid., 83–84.

23. Ibid., 84.

24. Ibid., 86.

25. Ibid., 87–88. There is also some question about the overall *quality* of the care rendered to the poor. Over half the Medicaid population is seen by only 16 percent of all physicians. Moreover, those physicians with large Medicaid populations were less frequently affiliated with hospitals. See Karen Davis, Marsha Gold, and Diane Makuc, "Access to Health Care for the Poor: Does the Gap Remain?" *Annual Review of Public Health* 1981:3.

26. See, among others, Illich's *Medical Nemesis* or Rick Carlson's *The End of Medicine* (New York: John Wiley and Sons, 1975) for examples of a nihilist approach to medical care.

27. David E. Rogers, Robert J. Blendon, and Thomas W. Maloney, "Who Needs Medicaid?" *New England Journal of Medicine* 307 (1982): 13, 16.

28. Jack Hadley, *More Health Care, Better Health? An Economic Analysis of Mortality Rates* (Washington, D.C.: Urban Institute Press, 1982), 2–3.

29. National Center for Health Statistics, *Health, United States, 1981.* Department of Health and Human Services (Washington, D.C.: Government Printing Office, 1981), 112.

30. President's Commission, *Securing Access,* 55.

31. *Containing Medical Care Costs Through Market Forces, A Congressional Budget Office Study,* May 1982: 26.

32. *National Data Book and Guide to Sources, Statistical Abstract of the United States, 1984,* U.S. Department of Commerce, Bureau of the Census (Washington, D.C.: U.S. Government Printing Office, 1983), 102.

33. Henry J. Aaron and William B. Schwartz, *The Painful Prescription: Rationing Hospital Care* (Washington, D.C.: Brookings Institute, 1984), 135. By contrast Victor Fuchs is one of a few who is clear that we are now rationing health care and always have been. See his "The 'Rationing' of Medical Care," *New England Journal of Medicine* 311 (December 13, 1984): 1572–1573. See also David Mechanic, "Cost Containment and the Quality of Medical Care: Rationing Strategies in an Era of Constrained Cost," *Milbank Memorial Fund Quarterly* 63 (1985): 453–475.

34. Arthur L. Caplan of the Hastings Center, among others, does not believe the case has been made yet for rationing (personal communication). See also Marcia Angell, "Cost Containment and the U.S. Physician," *Journal of the American Medical Association* 254,

no. 9 (September 6, 1985): 1203–1207, who claims that the involvement of physicians in rationing is "premature."

35. Willard Gaylin of the Hastings Center, among others, advocates this position.

36. Garrett Hardin, "The Tragedy of the Commons," *Science* 162 (December 13, 1968): 1243. This essay should be required reading for every student of distributive justice.

37. William Blythe, "Changing Perspectives of the End-Stage Renal Disease Program," *North Carolina Medical Journal* (June 1984): 404.

38. Brian Abel-Smith, "Who is the Odd Man Out? The Experience of Western Europe in Containing the Costs of Health Care," *Milbank Memorial Fund Quarterly* 63, no. 1 (1985).

39. For a masterful exposition of Adam Smith in relation to Rousseau and human needs, see Michael Ignatieff, *The Needs of Strangers* (New York: Viking Press, 1985), 105ff.

2. ETHICAL INDIVIDUALISM

1. Philip Slater, *The Pursuit of Loneliness: American Culture at the Breaking Point*, rev. ed. (Boston: Beacon Press, 1976), xiii–xiv. See also *Habits of the Heart* by Robert Bellah, et al. (Berkeley, Calif.: University of California Press, 1985), especially the section "Mythic Individualism," 144–147.

2. The name "Adam" in Genesis is simply the Hebrew word for "man" in the generic sense. Like the Adam of biblical mythology, the American in the parable thinks of himself as not only having dominion over nature but (wrongly) as also the originator of his moral precepts. Adam's original sin and the American's failing have a common motif—the hubris of moral invention that denies previous relatedness, Adam's relatedness to God and the American's to his former neighbors.

3. Ralph Waldo Emerson, "Self-Reliance," in *The Complete Writings of Ralph Waldo Emerson*, vol. 1 (New York: Wm. H. Wise, 1929), 139.

4. See Kass' "Regarding the End of Medicine and the Pursuit of Health," *The Public Interest* 40 (Summer 1975): 11–42; Knowles' "The Responsibility of the Individual," in *Doing Better and Feeling Worse: Health in the United States*, ed. J. H. Knowles (New York:

W. W. Norton, 1977); and Illich's *Medical Nemesis: The Expropriation of Health.*

5. In its Constitution, the World Health Organization defined "health" as not merely the absence of disease but "a state of complete physical, mental, and social well-being." *WHO: Basic Documents,* 2d. ed. (Geneva: World Health Organization, 1976), 1.

6. American Medical Association, *Code of Medical Ethics, 1847* (New York: H. Ludwig and Co., 1848). A good place to find the 1847 "Code" as well as subsequent codes and statements of principles is the appendix to volume 4 of *The Encyclopedia of Bioethics,* ed. Warren T. Reich (New York: The Free Press, 1978). 1737-1746.

7. *Encyclopedia of Bioethics,* 1739.

8. Ibid., 1750-1754.

9. Ibid., 1751.

10. *Opinions and Reports of the Judicial Council, American Medical Association* (1971), 53.

11. The 1980 "Principles" was adopted by the AMA House of Delegates at annual meeting, July 22, 1980. A full statement can be found in *Medical Ethics,* ed. Natalie Abrams and Michael Buckner (Cambridge, Mass.: MIT Press, 1983), 641-642.

12. See Murdoch's *The Sovereignty of Good* (London: Routledge and Kegan Paul, 1970), 1-45, where she argues that too much weight is given to choice and too little to "the prior work of attention" in moral theory.

13. For an excellent effort to justify this aspect of human morality on theoretical grounds, see Stanley Hauerwas and David Burrell's "From System to Story: An Alternative Pattern for Rationality in Ethics," in Hauerwas' *Truthfulness and Tragedy* (Notre Dame, Ind.: University of Notre Dame Press, 1977), 15-39.

14. Judith J. Thomson, "A Defense of Abortion," *Philosophy and Public Affairs* 1 (1971); 47-66.

15. This discussion of the lack of consent and its implications is drawn from Harmon L. Smith and Larry R. Churchill's *Professional Ethics and Primary Care Medicine* (Durham, N.C.: Duke University Press, 1986) 49-50.

16. David Kinzer, in "Care of the Poor Revisited," *Inquiry* 21 (Spring 1984): 12, puts the problem succinctly in terms of the unwillingness of some physicians to sign on for Medicaid: "You can't neglect patients you never see."

17. Rosalind Williams, "Two Kinds of Ethics," *The New York Times.* November 8, 1981.

18. Thomas H. Murray, "Ethics and Health Care Allocation," *Public Law Forum* 4, no. 1 (1984): 47.

19. This distinction between "identified" and "statistical" lives was introduced by Thomas Schelling, "The Life You Save May Be Your Own," in *Problems in Public Expenditure Analysis,* ed. Samuel B. Chase, Jr. (Washington, D.C.: Brookings Institute, 1966), 129–130.

20. A more complete account of the technical and policy developments surrounding hemodialysis can be found in Arthur L. Caplan's "How Should Values Count in the Allocation of New Technologies in Health Care?" in Bayer, Caplan, and Daniels' *In Search of Equity,* 99–122.

21. Jonathan Glover, *Causing Death and Saving Lives* (London: Pelican, 1977), 291.

22. Stanley Milgram, *Obedience to Authority: An Experimental View* (London: Harper & Row, 1974). Milgram's methods of gaining his data are themselves a case study of disregard for ethics in the use of human subjects.

23. See Roger Wertheimer's "Understanding the Abortion Argument," in *The Problem of Abortion,* 2d. ed., ed. Joel Feinberg (Belmont, Calif.: Wadsworth, 1984), 55–61.

24. Glover, *Causing Death and Saving Lives,* 292.

25. Alexis de Tocqueville, *Democracy in America,* vol. 2, trans. Henry Reeve (New York: Schocken Books, 1961), 120.

26. Ibid.

3. PERCEPTIONS OF JUSTICE

1. See, for example, the articles by Tom Beauchamp and Ruth Faden, Nora Bell, and Norman Daniels in *The Journal of Medicine and Philosophy* 4, no. 2 (1979), all of which, in very different ways, draw upon Rawls' *A Theory of Justice.*

2. John Rawls, *A Theory of Justice* (Cambridge, Mass.: Harvard University Press, 1971), 11.

3. Ibid., 60. Rawls gives a full statement of these principles on pp. 302–303.

4. Ibid., 302.

5. John Locke, *Second Treatise of Government* (1690), ed. C. B. MacPherson, (Indianapolis, Ind.: Hackett, 1980), 8–14.

6. Ibid., 52.

7. Ibid., 53.

8. George Parkin Grant, *English-Speaking Justice* (Notre Dame, Ind.: University of Notre Dame Press, 1985), 44.

9. Ibid.

10. Robert Nozick, *Anarchy, State, and Utopia* (New York: Basic Books, 1974), 149.

11. Ibid., 153.

12. Ibid.

13. Ibid., 32–33.

14. The individualistic assumption of both Rawls and Nozick was first brought to my attention by Alasdair MacIntyre in *After Virtue* (Notre Dame, Ind.: University of Notre Dame Press, 1981), 233, "Thus Rawls and Nozick articulate with great power a shared view which envisages entry into social life as—at least ideally—the voluntary act of at least potentially rational individuals with prior interest who have to ask the question 'What kind of social contract with others is it reasonable for me to enter into'?"

15. Aristotle, *Politics*, 1253a, in *The Basic Works of Aristotle*, ed. Richard McKeon (New York: Random House, 1941), 1129–1130.

16. Rawls, *A Theory of Justice*, 520.

17. Ibid., 522ff.

18. Michael J. Sandel, *Liberalism and the Limits of Justice* (Cambridge: Cambridge University Press, 1982), 150.

19. Ibid.

20. The seminal twentieth-century article on the ideal observer is Roderick Firth's "Ethical Absolutism and the Ideal Observer," *Philosophy and Phenomenological Research* 12 (1952).

21. See Rawls, *A Theory of Justice*, 184ff.

22. Immanuel Kant, *Foundations of the Metaphysics of Morals* (1785), trans. L. W. Beck (Indianapolis, Ind.: Bobbs-Merrill, 1956).

23. Kurt Baier, *The Moral Point of View: A Rational Basis of Ethics* (New York: Random House, 1965), 96, 107.

24. Rawls, *A Theory of Justice*, 185–186.

25. Adam Smith's use of the "impartial spectator" is the most extensive and insightful in Western moral theory and does not

succumb to the individualism of the contemporary uses of the "ideal observer." Smith's concept of sympathy is, as I argue later in the chapter, a link to a more realistic view of self and society.

26. Rawls, *A Theory of Justice*, 522.

27. Sandel, *Liberalism and the Limits of Justice*, 178.

28. Leon Kass, *Toward a More Natural Science: Biology and Human Affairs* (New York: The Free Press, 1985), 293.

29. See the brilliant essay by Erwin W. Strauss, "The Upright Posture," in his *Phenomenological Psychology*, trans. in part by Erling Eng (London: Tavistock, 1966), 137–165.

30. Kass, *Toward a More Natural Science*, 315.

31. Maurice Merleau-Ponty, *Phenomenology of Perception*, trans. by Colin Smith (London: Routledge and Kegan Paul, 1962), 362.

32. Adam Smith, *The Theory of Moral Sentiments*, (1759) ed. D. Raphael and A. Macfie (Oxford: Clarendon Press, 1976), 9.

33. Ibid., 10.

34. Ibid.

35. Ibid., 9.

36. Ibid., 112, emphasis added.

37. D. Raphael and A. Macfie, "Introduction," *The Theory of Moral Sentiments*, 1–25.

38. Elmer Sprague, "Adam Smith," *The Encyclopedia of Philosophy*, vol. 7, ed. Paul Edwards (New York: MacMillan, 1967), 462. A similar criticism is made by Max Scheler in his remarks on the inadequacies of the "ethics of sympathy" in *The Nature of Sympathy*, trans. Peter Heath (New Haven, Conn.: Yale University Press, 1954), 5–6. Scheler's position is actually more closely aligned to Smith than he realized.

39. Smith, *Theory of Moral Sentiments*, 88.

40. See, for example, David Hume's *An Enquiry Concerning the Principles of Morals* (1777) (La Salle, Ill.: Open Court, 1966), 54, n. 1. "It is needless to ask why we have humanity, or a fellow-feeling with others. It is sufficient that this is experienced to be a principle of human nature." Likewise, Bishop Joseph Butler in his first *Sermon* (1726) says, "It is as manifest that we are made for society, and to promote the happiness of it, as that we were intended to the care of our own life, and health, and private good."

41. H. Richard Niebuhr, *The Responsible Self* (New York: Harper & Row, 1963), 71.

42. Ibid., 73.

43. Louis Dumont, *Homo Hierarchicus: The Caste System and Its Implication,* trans. Mark Sainsbury, Louis Dumont, and Basio Gulati (Chicago: University of Chicago Press, 1980).

4. PRINCIPLES OF JUSTICE

1. Ronald Dworkin, *Taking Rights Seriously* (Cambridge, Mass.: Harvard University Press, 1977), xi. This discussion of rights as absolutes is adopted from an earlier discussion by Larry R. Churchill and José Jorge Simán, "Abortion and the Rhetoric of Individual Rights," *Hastings Center Report* 12 (February 1982): 9-12.

2. Quoted in Stanley I. Benn, "Rights," in *Encyclopedia of Philosophy,* vol. 7 (New York: Macmillan and Free Press, 1967), 197.

3. Joel Feinberg, *Social Philosophy* (Englewood Cliffs, N.J.: Prentice-Hall, 1973), 58-67.

4. Nozick, *Anarchy, State, and Utopia,* 233-235.

5. For this argument I am indebted to Howard Brody, "The Rights-as-Trumps Analogy," *Hastings Center Report* 12, no. 5 (October 1982): 45.

6. Robert Sade, "Medical Care as a Right: A Refutation," *New England Journal of Medicine* 285, no. 23, (December 2, 1971): 1288ff.

7. "Market Justice" is a term used by Dan E. Beauchamp in "Public Health as Social Justice," *Inquiry* 13, no. 1 (March 1976): 4-6.

8. An extended version of these arguments against the market model of justice in health care can be found in Smith and Churchill, *Professional Ethics and Primary Care Medicine,* 93-96.

9. Victor Sidel, "The Right to Health Care: An International Perspective," in *Bioethics and Human Rights: A Reader for Health Professionals,* ed. E. L. Bandman and B. Bandman (Boston: Little, Brown, 1978), 347. A case similar to Sidel's is made by Paul F. Camenisch, "The Right to Health Care: A Contractual Approach," *Soundings* 62, no. 3 (Fall 1979), 293-310.

10. It is useful to remember that the term 'profession' was originally a vow or pledge made upon entrance to a religious order. Though tainted by the contemporary contrast with 'amateur' and associated with "doing it for money" (evoking unsavory images), 'professional' still implies a calling in which the public good is placed above private

gain, and thereby, public trust is confirmed. It is striking that while recent medical codes have scrupulously avoided any mention of medicine's indebtedness and subsequent obligation to society, nurses have made this quite explicit. The American Nurses' Association's *Code for Nurses* says, "The use of the title *registered nurse* is granted by the state governments for the protection of the public. Use of that title carries with it the responsibility to act in the public interest." *Code for Nurses with Interpretive Statements* (Kansas City, Mo.: American Nurses' Association, 1985), 15.

11. James Childress, "A Right to Health Care," *Journal of Medicine and Philosophy* 4, no. 2 (June 1979): 134.

12. Nozick, *Anarchy, State, and Utopia*, 235.

13. See Engelhardt's Shattuck Lecture of 1984 "Allocating Scarce Medical Resources and the Availability of Organ Transplantation: Some Moral Presuppositions," *New England Journal of Medicine* 311 (July 5, 1984): 66–71, and his "Personal Health Care or Preventive Care: Distributing Scarce Medical Resources," *Soundings* 63, no. 3 (Fall 1980): 234–256.

14. Engelhardt, Shattuck Lecture, 70.

15. Engelhardt, "Personal Health Care or Preventive Care," 248.

16. Ibid., 245.

17. Ibid., 249.

18. Engelhardt, Shattuck Lecture, 70–71.

19. Engelhardt, *The Foundations of Bioethics* (New York: Oxford University Press, 1986), 70. Some of Engelhardt's earlier work was more balanced and had a place for sociality. See, for example, "Moral Autonomy and the Polis: A Response to Gerald Dworkin and Gregory Vlastos," in *Morals, Science and Sociality,* ed. H. T. Engelhardt and Daniel Callahan (Hastings-on-Hudson, New York: Institute of Society, Ethics, and the Life Sciences, 1978), 202–214.

20. Ibid., 353ff.

21. Harold Laski, *The Decline of Liberalism,* the L. T. Hobbhouse Memorial Trust Lecture No. 10, (London: Oxford University Press, 1940), 22.

22. Henry E. Sigerist, "Social Medicine," *The Yale Review* 27, no. 3 (Spring 1938): 462–481, reprinted in *Moral Problems in Medicine,* ed. Samuel Gorowitz, et al. (Engelwood Cliffs, N.J.: Prentice-Hall, 1976), 468.

23. George Silver, "Reply to Professor Bryant," *International Journal of Health Services* 7 (1977): 724. See also Leonard Syme

and Ira Berkman, "Social Class Susceptibility and Sickness," *American Journal of Epidemiology* 104, no. 1 (July 1976): 1–8, who indicated that persons in lower class groups have higher morbidity and mortality rates of almost every disease and illness. On the relationship between socioeconomic status and health care, see Patrick W. Conover, "Social Class and Chronic Illness," *International Journal of Health Services* 3, no. 3 (1973): 357–368.

24. Engelhardt, Shattuck Lecture, 71.

25. See William Ryan, *Blaming the Victim* (New York: Vintage Books, 1971), especially pp. 156–163.

26. Dan E. Beauchamp, "Public Health as Social Justice," 5.

27. Robert M. Veatch, "Voluntary Risks to Health: The Ethical Issues," *Journal of the American Medical Association* 243 (January 4, 1980): 50–55. See also Veatch's *A Theory of Medical Ethics* (New York: Basic Books, 1981) 280.

28. Mark Siegler, "A Physician's Perspective on a Right to Health Care," *Journal of the American Medical Association* 244 (October 3, 1980): 1591–1596.

29. Peter Singer, "Freedoms and Utilities in the Distribution of Health Care," in *Ethics and Health Policy,* ed. Robert Veatch and Roy Branson (Cambridge, Mass.: Ballinger, 1976), 175–193.

30. Charles Fried, "An Analysis of 'Equality' and 'Rights' in Medical Care" in *Ethical Issues in Modern Medicine,* 2d. ed., ed. John Arras and Robert Hunt (Palo Alto, Calif.: Mayfield, 1983), 494ff.

31. Ibid.

32. Paul Camenisch, "The Right to Health Care: A Contractual Approach," 307.

33. Ibid., 308.

34. Norman Daniels, *Just Health Care* (Cambridge: Cambridge University Press, 1985), 19–58. My basic disagreement with Daniels is not in his conclusions, but in his premises. He, like many others, believes it is sufficient to arrive at basic principles of allocation and neglects the social sentiments to which principles of justice appeal.

35. Amy Gutmann, "For and Against Equal Access to Health Care," in *In Search of Equity,* ed. Ronald Bayer, Arthur Kaplan, and Norman Daniels (New York: Plenum Press, 1983), 43–67.

36. Tom Beauchamp and Ruth Faden, "The Right to Health and the Right to Health Care," *Journal of Medicine and Philosophy* 4, no. 2 (June 1979): 121–122.

37. Philip R. Lee and Albert R. Jonsen, "The Right to Health

Care," editorial, *American Review of Respiratory Disease* 109 (1974): 591-592.

38. President's Commission, *Securing Access*, 19ff.

39. See, for example, Robert P. Rhodes, "Optimizing Health: Why Equality of Access to Health Care Based on Need Leads to Injustice," in *Respect and Care in Medical Ethics*, ed. David H. Smith (Lanham, Mass.: University Press of America, 1984), 187-213. Rhodes seems to believe in a radical and irremediable relativity in the definition of needs, claiming that "most are difficult for patient or physician to identify" (p. 189). Here he seems to confuse 'health', which is no doubt a "contested concept," with health needs, which we routinely depend on the expertise of physicians to define.

40. The phrase "the needs of strangers" is borrowed from Michael Ignatieff's book by the same name, cited earlier.

41. See Daniel Callahan's "Minimalist Ethics," *Hastings Center Report* 11, no. 5 (October 1981): 19-25. Callahan correctly argues that a minimalist ethics confuses useful principles for government regulations and civil liberties with the broader requirements for a moral life.

42. For a good discussion of the concepts of 'community' and 'society', see Joseph R. Gusfield's *Community: A Critical Response* (New York: Harper & Row, 1975).

43. John Macmurray, *Persons in Relation* (London: Faber and Faber, 1961), 153.

5. THE PHYSICIAN'S ROLE AND POLICIES OF RATIONING

1. Lester Thurow, "Learning to Say 'No'," *New England Journal of Medicine* 311, no. 24 (December 13, 1984), 1571.

2. Ibid.

3. Ibid.

4. Marcia Angell, "Cost Containment and the Physician," 1203.

5. Norman Levinsky, "The Doctor's Master," *New England Journal of Medicine* 31, no. 24 (December 13, 1984), 1573. See also Robert Veatch, "A Novel Proposal," *Massachusetts Medicine* 4, no. 1 (1986), 45ff.

6. Howard Hiatt, "Protecting the Medical Commons: Who is Responsible?" *New England Journal of Medicine* 293 (July 31, 1975), 241. See also George Agich and Charles Begley, "Some Problems

with Pro-Competition Reforms," *Social Science and Medicine* 21, no. 6 (1985). This conviction is now a part of the official AMA stance; see the Judicial Council's "Opinions" of 1984 (Chicago: American Medical Association), 3.

7. Roger W. Evans, "Health Care Technology and the Inevitability of Resource Allocating and Rationing Decisions," part 2, *Journal of the American Medical Association* 249, no. 16 (April 29, 1983); 2208.

8. Reinhold Niebuhr, *Moral Man and Immoral Society* (New York: Charles Scribner's Sons, 1960), 248-249.

9. Cited in David Mechanic, "Ethics, Justice, and Medical Care Systems," in *Medical Ethics and Social Change*, ed. Barnard Barber, vol. 437 of *Annals of the American Association of Political and Social Science* (May 1978), 77.

10. Levinsky, "The Doctor's Master," quoting Howard Hiatt, 1574.

11. See Larry R. Churchill, Stanley Hauerwas, and Harmon L. Smith, "Medical Care for the Poor: Finite Resources, Infinite Need," *Health Progress* 66, no. 10 (December 1985): 32-35.

12 Leon Kass, "The Case for Mortality," *The American Scholar* 52, no. 2 (Spring 1983): 187. This essay is reprinted in *Toward a More Natural Science.*

13. Rudolf Klein, "Rationing Health Care," *British Medical Journal* 289 (July 21, 1984): 144.

14. Resource Allocation Working Party, *Sharing Resources for Health in England: Report of the Resource Allocation Working Party* (London, DHSS, 1976), 8.

15. Ibid., 9-10.

16. Henry J. Aaron and William B. Schwartz, *The Painful Prescription: Rationing Hospital Care* (Washington, D.C.: Brookings Institute, 1984), 97-99.

17. Ibid., 101-102.

18. I owe these considerations to many conversations with the Fellows of the King's Fund College, London, during the summer of 1985.

19. E. Harvey Estes (Chairman), et al., *A Manpower Policy for Primary Health Care*, Institute of Medicine, National Academy of Sciences (1978), IOM Publication 78-02, p. 1.

20. Milton Friedman, *Capitalism and Freedom* (Chicago: University of Chicago Press, 1962), 187-188.

21. *Organ Transplantation,* Report of the Task Force on Organ Transplantation (Washington, D.C.: U.S. Department of Health and Human Services, April 1986), 9, 11, 102–104.

22. Here I am indebted to Paul James and Michael Richardson, two of my former students with whom I have discussed the issues of allocation and ordering of priorities at some length. Also, I leave aside altogether questions of medical research and which areas of research should be funded.

23. Here I have drawn from James Childress' discussion in *Priorities in Biomedical Ethics* (Philadelphia: Westminster, 1981), 82–83.

24. Paul Starr, "The Politics of Therapeutic Nihilism," *Hastings Center Report* 6, no. 5 (October 1976), 29.

25. Michael Michaelson, "The Coming Medical War," in *Readings on Ethical and Social Issues in Biomedicine,* in Richard W. Wertz (Engelwood Cliffs, N.J.: Prentice-Hall, 1973), 269–285.

26. Peter Townsend and Nick Davidson, *Inequalities in Health* (London: Penguin, 1982).

27. Danielle A. Dolenc and Charles J. Daugherty, "DRGs: The Counterrevolution in Financing Health Care," *Hastings Center Report* 15, no. 3 (June 1985): 19–29.

28. See John K. Iglehart, "Medicare Begins Prospective Payment of Hospitals," *New England Journal of Medicine* 308 (1983): 1428–1432, and B. C. Vladek, "Medicare Hospital Payment by Diagnosis-Related Groups," *Annals of Internal Medicine* 100 (1984): 573–591.

29. B. E. Spivey, "The Relation Between Hospital Management and Medical Staff Under a Prospective Payment System," *New England Journal of Medicine* 310 (April 12, 1984): 984–986.

30. For a good discussion of the tensions DRGs may exacerbate within the physician's role, see Haavi Morreim, "The MD and the DRG," *Hastings Center Report* 15, no. 3 (July 1985): 30–38.

31. Victor R. Fuchs, *The Health Economy* (Cambridge, Mass.: Harvard University Press, 1986), 353.

32. See Robert J. Blendon, et al., "Uncompensated Care by Hospitals or Public Insurance for the Poor: Does It Make a Difference?" *New England Journal of Medicine* 312 (1986): 1160–1163.

CONCLUSION

1. David Wessel, "Transplants Increase and So Do Disputes Over Who Pays Bills," *Wall Street Journal,* vol. 73, April 12, 1984, pp. 1, 24.

2. *Raleigh News and Observer,* June 13, 1985.
3. See, for example, Robert Bellah, et al. *Habits of the Heart: Individualism and Commitment in American Life;* William M. Sullivan, *Reconstructing Public Philosophy* (Berkeley, Calif.: University of California Press, 1982).
4. William M. Sullivan, *Reconstructing Public Philosophy,* 157.

Selected Bibliography

Aaron, Henry J., and William B. Schwartz. *The Painful Prescription: Rationing Hospital Care.* Washington, D.C.: Brookings Institute, 1984.

Abel-Smith, Brian. "Who is the Odd Man Out? The Experience of Western Europe in Containing the Costs of Health Care." *Milbank Memorial Fund Quarterly* 63 (1985).

Agich, George J., and Charles E. Begley. "Some Problems with Pro-Competition Reforms." *Social Science and Medicine* 21, no. 6 (1985).

Almy, Thomas P. "The Role of the Primary Care Physician in the Health-Care 'Industry'." *New England Journal of Medicine* 304 (January 22, 1981).

American Medical Association. *Code of Medical Ethics 1847.* New York: H. Ludwig and Co., 1848.

————. "Principles of Medical Ethics," adopted by the House of Delegates, July 22, 1980.

American Nurses Association. *Code for Nurses with Interpretive Statements.* Kansas City, Mo.: American Nurses Association, 1985.

Angell, Marcia. "Cost Containment and the U.S. Physician." *Journal of the American Medical Association* 254 (September 6, 1985).

Annas, George J. "Adam Smith in the Emergency Room." *Hastings Center Report* 15 (August 1985).

Aristotle. *Politics.* In *The Basic Works of Aristotle,* edited by Richard McKeon. New York: Random House, 1941.

Arras, John. "The Neoconservative Health Strategy." In *Ethical Issues in Modern Medicine,* 2d ed., edited by John Arras and Robert Hunt. Palo Alto, Calif.: Mayfield, 1983.

Arras, John, and Andrew Jameton. "Medical Individualism and the Right to Health Care." In *Intervention and Reflection: Basic Issues in Medical Ethics,* edited by Ronald Munson. Belmont, Calif.: Wadsworth, 1979.

Bayer, Ronald. "Getting to the Heart of Things" (Guest Editorial). *The New Physician* (April 1985).

Bayer, Ronald, Arthur Caplan, and Norman Daniels, eds. *In Search of Equity: Health Needs and the Health Care System.* New York: Plenum Press, 1983.

Beauchamp, Dan E. "Public Health as Social Justice." *Inquiry* 13 (March 1976).

————. "Community: The Neglected Tradition of Public Health." *Hastings Center Report* 15 (December 1985).

Beauchamp, Tom L., and James F. Childress. *Principles of Biomedical Ethics.* 2d ed. New York: Oxford University Press, 1983.

Bellah, Robert, Richard Madson, William Sullivan, Ann Swidler, and Steven Tipton. *Habits of the Heart: Individualism and Commitment in American Life.* Berkeley, Calif.: University of California Press, 1985.

Benn, Stanley I. "Rights." In *The Encyclopedia of Philosophy,* vol. 7, edited by Paul Edwards. New York: MacMillan and Free Press, 1967.

Blackstone, William. "Health Care as a Right." *Georgia Law Review* 10 (1976).

Blendon, Robert J., et al. "Uncompensated Care by Hospitals or Public Insurance for the Poor: Does It Make a Difference?" *New England Journal of Medicine* 314 (May 1, 1986).

Blendon, Robert J., and Drew E. Altman. "Public Attitudes About Health Care: A Lesson in National Schizophrenia." *New England Journal of Medicine* 311 (August 30, 1984).

Bluestone, Naomi. "Don't be a Litterbug: Dispose of Health Properly." *New England Journal of Medicine* 293 (July 1975).

Blythe, William. "Changing Perspectives of the End-Stage Renal Disease Program." *North Carolina Medical Journal* (June 1984).

Boyle, Joseph F. "Should We Learn to Say 'No'?" *Journal of the American Medical Association* 252 (1984).

Brazda, J., ed. "Perspectives: Who Will Care for the Uninsured?" *Washington Report on Medicine and Health* 36 (September 27, 1982).

Brazil, Percy. "Cost Effective Care is Better Care." *Hastings Center Report* 16 (February 1986).

Brody, Howard. *Ethical Decisions in Medicine.* 2d ed. Boston: Little, Brown, 1981.

Butler, Bishop Joseph. *Sermons* (1726). In *Ethical Theories: A Book of Readings,* 2d ed., edited by A. I. Melden. Englewood Cliffs, N.J.: Prentice-Hall, 1955.

Callahan, Daniel. "Minimalist Ethics." *Hastings Center Report* 11 (October 1981).

Camenisch, Paul F. "The Right to Health Care: A Contractual Approach." *Soundings* (Fall 1979).

Campbell, Alastair. *Medicine, Health and Justice.* Edinburgh: Churchill Livingstone, 1981.

Caplan, Arthur L. "Kidneys, Ethics and Politics: Lessons of the ESRD Program." *Journal of Health Politics, Policy and Law* 6 (Fall 1981).

Childress, James. "Citizen and Physician: Harmonious or Conflicting Responsibilities?" *Journal of Medicine and Philosophy* 2 (December 1977).

————. "A Right to Health Care." *Journal of Medicine and Philosophy* 4 (June 1979).

————. *Priorities in Biomedical Ethics.* Philadelphia: The Westminster Press, 1981.

Churchill, Larry, Stanley Hauerwas, and Harmon Smith. "Medical Care for the Poor: Finite Resources, Infinite Need." *Health Progress* 66 (December 1985).

Conover, Patrick W. "Social Class and Chronic Illness." *International Journal of Health Services* 3 (1973).

Couto, Richard. "Property, Pinmakers and Physicians: Liberal Myths and American Health Care." *Soundings* 62 (Fall 1979).

Current Medical Opinions of the Judicial Council of the American Medical Association. Chicago: The American Medical Association, 1984.

Daniels, Norman. *Just Health Care.* Cambridge: Cambridge University Press, 1985.

————. "Why Saying No to Patients in the United States is So Hard." *New England Journal of Medicine* 314 (May 22, 1986).

Davis, Karen. "The Impact of Inflation and Unemployment on Health Care of Low Income Families." In *Health: A Victim or Cause of Inflation,* edited by M. Zubcoff. New York: Prodist Press, 1976.

Davis, Karen, Marsha Gold, and Diane Makuc. "Access to Health Care for the Poor: Does the Gap Remain?" *Annual Review of Public Health* (1981).

Davis, Karen, and Diane Rowland. "Uninsured and Underserved: Inequities in Health Care in the United States." *Milbank Memorial Quarterly* 61 (1983).

Dolenc, Danielle A., and Charles J. Daugherty. "DRGs: The Counter-revolution in Financing Health Care." *Hastings Center Report* 15 (June 1985).

Dworkin, Ronald. *Taking Rights Seriously.* Cambridge, Mass.: Harvard University Press, 1977.

Dyck, Arthur J. *On Human Care.* Nashville, Tenn.: Abingdon, 1977.

Dyer, Allen R. "Patients, Not Costs, Come First." *Hastings Center Report* 16 (February 1986).

Emerson, Ralph Waldo. *The Complete Writings of Ralph Waldo Emerson.* New York: Wm. H. Wise, 1929.

Engelhardt, H. T. "Personal Health Care or Preventive Care: Distributing Scarce Medical Resources." *Soundings* 63 (Fall 1980).

————. "Shattuck Lecture—Allocating Scarce Medical Resources and the Availability of Organ Transplantation: Some Moral Presuppositions." *New England Journal of Medicine* 311 (July 5, 1984).

————. *The Foundations of Bioethics.* New York: Oxford University Press, 1986.

————, ed. "Rights to Health Care." *Journal of Medicine and Philosophy* 4, no. 2 (June 1979).

Engelhardt, H. T., and Daniel Callahan, eds. *Morals, Science and Sociality.* Hastings-on-Hudson, New York: Institute of Society, Ethics and Life Sciences, 1978.

Enthoven, Alain. *Health Plan.* Reading, Mass.: Addison-Wesley, 1980.

Estes, E. Harvey, et al. "A Manpower Policy for Primary Health Care." Washington, D.C.: Institute of Medicine, National Academy of Sciences, IOM Publication 78–02 (1978).

Evans, Roger W. "Health Care Technology and the Inevitability of Resource Allocation and Rationing Decisions." *Journal of the American Medical Association* 249 (1983).

Fein, Rashi. "On Achieving Access and Equity in Health Care." *Milbank Memorial Quarterly* 50 (1972).

Feinberg, Joel. *Social Philosophy.* Englewood Cliffs, N.J.: Prentice-Hall, 1973.

Firth, Roderick. "Ethical Absolutism and the Ideal Observer." *Philosophy and Phenomenological Research* 12 (1952).

Fletcher, Joseph. *Morals and Medicine.* Boston: Beacon Press, 1960.

Fried, Charles. "Rights and Health Care: Beyond Equity and Efficiency." *New England Journal of Medicine* 293 (July 31, 1975).

_____. "An Analysis of 'Equality' and 'Rights' in Medical Care." In *Ethical Issues in Modern Medicine*, 2d ed., edited by John Arras and Robert Hunt. Palo Alto, Calif.: Mayfield Publishing, 1983.

Friedman, Milton. *Capitalism and Freedom*. Chicago: University of Chicago Press, 1962.

Fuchs, Victor. *Who Shall Live? Health, Economics and Social Choice*. New York: Basic Books, 1974.

_____. "The 'Rationing' of Medical Care." *New England Journal of Medicine* 311 (December 13, 1984).

_____. *The Health Economy*. Cambridge, Mass.: Harvard University Press, 1986.

Fuller, Lon. "Two Principles of Human Association." In *Voluntary Associations*, edited by J. R. Pennock and J. W. Chapman. New York: Atherton Press, 1969.

Gerber, Alex. "Let's *Forget* About Equality of Care." *Prism* 3 (October 1975).

Gibson, Robert M., Daniel R. Waldo, and Katherine R. Levit. "National Health Expenditures, 1982." *Health Care Financing Review* 5 (Fall 1983).

Glover, Jonathan. *Causing Death and Saving Lives*. London: Pelican, 1977.

Goodin, Robert E. "Vulnerabilities and Responsibilities—An Ethical Defense of the Welfare State." *The American Political Science Review* 79 (September 1985).

Grant, George Parkin. *English-Speaking Justice*. Notre Dame, Ind.: Univeristy of Notre Dame Press, 1985.

Green, Ronald M. "Health Care and Justice in Contract Theory Perspective." In *Ethics and Health Policy*, edited by Robert Veatch and Roy Branson. Cambridge, Mass.: Ballinger, 1976.

Gusfield, Joseph R. *Community: A Critical Response*. New York: Harper & Row, 1975.

Gutmann, Amy. "For and Against Equal Access to Health Care." *Milbank Memorial Fund Quarterly* 59 (Fall 1981).

Hadley, Jack. *More Health Care, Better Health? An Economic Analysis of Mortality Rates*. Washington, D.C.: Urban Institute Press, 1982.

Halper, Thomas. "Life and Death in a Welfare State: End-Stage Renal Disease in the United Kingdom." *Milbank Memorial Fund Quarterly* 63 (Winter 1985).

Hardin, Garrett, "The Tragedy of the Commons." *Science* 162 (December 13, 1968).

Harron, Frank, John Burnside, and Tom Beauchamp. *Health and Human Values.* New Haven, Conn.: Yale University Press, 1983.

Hauerwas, Stanley. *Truthfulness and Tragedy.* Notre Dame, Ind.: University of Notre Dame Press, 1977.

Hauerwas, Stanley, and Alasdair MacIntyre. *Revisions: Changing Perspectives in Moral Philosophy.* Notre Dame, Ind.: University of Notre Dame Press, 1983.

Hiatt, Howard H. "Protecting the Medical Commons: Who is Responsible?" *New England Journal of Medicine* 293 (July 31, 1975).

Honigsbaum, Frank. *The Division in British Medicine.* London: Kogan Page, 1979.

Hume, David. *An Enquiry Concerning the Principles of Morals* (1777). LaSalle, Ill.: Open Court, 1966.

Ignatieff, Michael. *The Needs of Strangers.* New York: Viking Press, 1985.

Iglehart, John K. "Medicare Begins Prospective Payment of Hospitals." *New England Journal of Medicine* 308 (June 9, 1983).

————. "Medical Care for the Poor—A Growing Problem." *New England Journal of Medicine* 313 (July 4, 1985).

Illich, Ivan. *Medical Nemesis: The Expropriation of Health.* New York: Pantheon Books, 1976.

Jonsen, Albert R., and Andrew L. Jameton. "Social and Political Responsibilities of Physicians." *Journal of Medicine and Philosophy* 2 (December 1977).

Judicial Council, American Medical Association. "Current Opinions." Chicago: American Medical Association, 1984.

Kant, Immanuel. *Foundations of the Metaphysics of Morals* (1785). Translated by L. W. Beck. Indianapolis, Ind.: Bobbs-Merrill, 1956.

Kass, Leon R. "Regarding the End of Medicine and the Pursuit of Health." *The Public Interest* 40 (Summer 1975).

————. *Toward a More Natural Science: Biology and Human Affairs.* New York: The Free Press, 1985.

Kinzer, David. "Care of the Poor Revisited." *Inquiry* 21 (Spring 1984).

Klein, Rudolf. *The Politics of the National Health Service.* London: Longman, Harlon, 1983.

————. "Rationing Health Care." *British Medical Journal* 289 (July 21, 1984).

Knowles, John H., ed. *Doing Better and Feeling Worse: Health Care in the United States.* New York: W. W. Norton, 1977.

Kosa, John, Aaron Antonovsky, and Irving Zola. *Poverty and Health: A Sociological Analysis.* Cambridge, Mass.: Harvard University Press, 1969.

Laski, Harold. *The Decline of Liberalism, L. T. Hobbhouse Memorial Trust Lecture No. 10.* London: Oxford University Press, 1940.

Leaf, Alexander. "The Doctor's Dilemma—and Society's Too." *New England Journal of Medicine* 310 (March 15, 1984).

Lee, Philip R., and Albert Jonsen. "The Right to Health Care." *American Review of Respiratory Disease* 109 (1974).

Lefton, Doug. *American Medical News* (April 20, 1984). "Public Hospital Limits Care to Tampa's Poor."

Levinsky, Norman. "The Doctor's Master." *New England Journal of Medicine* 311 (December 13, 1984).

Levin, M. E., and L. S. Levin. "Health Care for the Uninsured." *Business and Health* 1 (September 1984).

Locke, John. *Second Treatise of Government* (1690). Edited by C. B. MacPherson. Indianapolis, Ind.: Hackett, 1980.

Loewy, Erich H. "Cost Should Not Be A Factor In Medical Care." *New England Journal of Medicine* 302 (March 20, 1980).

Lukes, Steven. *Individualism.* New York: Harper & Row, 1973.

MacIntyre, Alasdair. "Egoism and Altruism." In *Encyclopedia of Philosophy,* vol. 2, edited by Paul Edwards. New York: MacMillan and The Free Press, 1967.

————. *After Virtue.* Notre Dame, Ind.: University of Notre Dame Press, 1981.

Macmurray, John. *Persons in Relation.* London: Faber and Faber, 1961.

Maynard, A., and A. Ludbrook. "Applying Resource Allocation Formula to Constituent Parts of the U.K." *Lancet* 1 (1980).

————. "Thirty Years of Fruitless Endeavor? An Analysis of Government Intervention in the Health Care Market." In *Health, Economics and Health Economics,* edited by Van der Goag and Perlman. New York: North Holland Publishing, 1981.

McCormick, Richard A. "Some Neglected Aspects of Moral Responsibility for Health." *Perspective in Biology and Medicine* (Autumn 1978).

McGinnis, J. "Recent Health Gains for Adults." *New England Journal of Medicine* 306 (1982).

Mechanic, David. "Rationing Health Care: Public Policy and the Medical Market Place." *Hastings Center Report* 6 (1976).

_____. "Ethics, Justice and Medical Care Systems." In *Medical Ethics and Social Change*, vol. 437 of *The Annals of the American Academy of Political and Social Science*, edited by Barnard Barber (May 1978).

_____. "Cost Containment and the Quality of Medical Care: Rationing Strategies in an Era of Constrained Cost." *Milbank Memorial Fund Quarterly* 63 (1985).

Menzel, Paul J. *Medical Costs, Moral Choices.* New Haven, Conn.: Yale University Press, 1983.

Merleau-Ponty, Maurice. *Phenomenology of Perception.* Translated by Colin Smith. London: Routledge and Kegan Paul, 1962.

Michaelson, Michael. "The Coming Medical War." In *Readings on Ethical and Social Issues in Biomedicine*, edited by Richard W. Wertz. Englewood Cliffs, N.J.: Prentice-Hall, 1973.

Milgram, Stanley. *Obedience to Authority: An Experimental View.* London: Harper & Row, 1974.

Miller, Frances H., and Graham Miller. "The Painful Prescription: A Procrustean Perspective. *New England Journal of Medicine* 314 (May 22, 1986).

Minogue, Kenneth. *The Liberal Mind.* New York: Random House, 1963.

Morison, Robert S. "Rights and Responsibilities: Redressing the Uneasy Balance." *Hastings Center Report* 4 (April 1974).

Morreim, E. Haavi. "Cost Containment: Issues of Moral Conflict and Justice for Physicians." *Theoretical Medicine* 6 (1985).

_____. "The MD and the DRG." *Hastings Center Report* 15 (July 1985).

Mundinger, Mary O'Neil. "Health Service Funding Cuts and the Declining Health of the Poor." *New England Journal of Medicine* 313 (July 4, 1985).

Murdoch, Iris. *The Sovereignty of Good.* London: Routledge and Kegan Paul, 1970.

Murray, Thomas H. "Ethics and Health Care Allocation." *Public Law Forum* 4 (1984).

National Center for Health Statistics, Department of Health and Human Services. *Health in the United States, 1981.* Washington, D.C.: U.S. Government Printing Office, 1981.

Niebuhr, H. Richard. *The Responsible Self.* New York: Harper & Row, 1963.

Niebuhr, Reinhold. *Moral Man and Immoral Society*. New York: Charles Scribner's Sons, 1960.

Nozick, Robert. *Anarchy, State and Utopia*. New York: Basic Books, 1974.

Outka, Gene. "Social Justice and Equal Access to Health Care." *Journal of Religious Ethics* 2 (1974).

President's Commission for the Study of Ethical Problems in Medicine and Biomedical and Behavioral Research. *Securing Access to Health Care*. Vol. 1. Washington, D.C.: U.S. Government Printing Office, 1983.

Preston, Thomas A. "The Artificial Heart and the Public Purse." *Medical World News* (September 10, 1984).

Rabkin, Mitchell T. "Control of Health-Care Costs, Targeting and Coordinating the Economic Incentives." *New England Journal of Medicine* 309 (October 20, 1983).

Radical Statistics Health Group. *In Defense of the NHS*. London, 1977.

Ramsey, Paul. *The Patient as Person: Explorations in Medical Ethics*. New Haven, Conn.: Yale University Press, 1970.

Rawls, John. *A Theory of Justice*. Cambridge, Mass.: Harvard University Press, 1971.

Relman, Arnold. "The Allocation of Medical Resources by Physicians." *Journal of American Education* 55 (February 1980).

————. "The New Medical-Industrial Complex." *New England Journal of Medicine* 303 (October 23, 1980).

Resource Allocation Working Party. *Sharing Resources for Health in England: Report of the Resource Allocation Working Party*. London: Department of Health and Social Services, 1976.

Reuben, David. "Learning Diagnostic Restraint." *New England Journal of Medicine* 310 (March 1, 1984).

Rhodes, Robert P. "Optimizing Health: Why Equality of Access to Health Care Based on Need Leads to Injustice." In *Respect and Care in Medical Ethics,* edited by David M. Smith. Lanham, Mass.: University Press of America, 1984.

Rogers, David E., Robert J. Blendon, and Thomas W. Maloney. "Who Needs Medicaid?" *New England Journal of Medicine* 307 (1982).

Rousseau, Jean Jacques. *The Social Contract* (1762). Translated by G. D. H. Cole. New York: E. P. Dutton, 1950.

Ryan, William. *Blaming the Victim*. New York: Vintage Books, 1971.

Sade, Robert. "Medical Care as a Right: A Refutation." *New England Journal of Medicine* 285 (December 2, 1971).

Sandel, Michael J. *Liberalism and the Limits of Justice.* Cambridge: Cambridge University Press, 1982.

Scheffler, R., et al. *Physicians and New Health Practitioners: Issues for the 1980's.* Institute of Medicine, National Academy of Sciences, 1979.

Schelling, Thomas. "The Life You Save May Be Your Own." In *Problems in Public Expenditure Analysis,* edited by Samuel B. Chase, Jr. Washington, D.C.: Brookings Institute, 1966.

Schrag, Brian. "Justice and the Justification of a Social Policy: The Distribution of Primary Care Physicians." *Social Science and Medicine* 17 (1983).

_____. "Social Obligations for Primary Care." In *Respect and Care in Medical Ethics,* edited by David H. Smith. Lanham, Md.: University Press of America, 1984.

Sidel, Victor. "The Right to Health Care: An International Perspective." In *Bioethics and Human Rights: A Reader for Health Professionals,* edited by E. L. Bandman and B. Bandman. Boston: Little, Brown, 1978.

Sidel, Victor W., and Ruth Sidel. *A Healthy State.* Rev. ed. New York: Pantheon Books, 1983.

Siegler, Mark. "A Physician's Perspective on a Right to Health Care." *Journal of the American Medical Association* 244 (October 3, 1980).

Sigerist, Henry E. "Social Medicine." *The Yale Review* 27 (Spring 1938). Reprinted in *Moral Problems in Medicine,* edited by Samuel Gorowitz, et al. Englewood Cliffs, N.J.: Prentice-Hall, 1976.

Silver, George. "Reply to Professor Bryant." *International Journal of Health Care.*" In *Ethics and Health Policy,* edited by Robert Veatch and Roy Branson. Cambridge, Mass.: Ballinger, 1976.

Slater, Philip. *The Pursuit of Loneliness: American Culture at the Breaking Point.* Rev. ed. Boston: Beacon Press, 1976.

Smith, Adam. *The Theory of Moral Sentiments* (1759). Edited by D. Raphael and A. Macfie. Oxford: Clarendon Press, 1976.

Smith, Harmon L., and Larry R. Churchill. *Professional Ethics and Primary Care Medicine: Beyond Dilemmas and Decorum.* Durham, N.C.: Duke University Press, 1986.

Spivey, B. E. "The Relation Between Hospital Management and

Medical Staff Under a Prospective Payment System." *New England Journal of Medicine* 310 (April 12, 1984).

Stackhouse, Max. *Creeds, Society and Human Rights: A Study in Three Cultures.* Grand Rapids, Mich.: Eerdmans, 1984.

Starr, Paul. "The Politics of Therapeutic Nihilism." *Hastings Center Report* 6 (October 1976).

_____. *The Social Transformation of American Medicine.* New York: Basic Books, 1982.

Strauss, Erwin W. "The Upright Posture." In *Phenomenological Psychology,* translated, in part, by Erling Eng. London: Tavistock, 1966.

Sullivan, William M. *Reconstructing Public Philosophy.* Berkeley, Calif.: University of California Press, 1982.

Syme, Leonard, and Ira Berkman. "Social Class, Susceptibility and Sickness." *American Journal of Epidemiology* 104 (1976).

Szasz, Thomas S. "The Right to Health." *Georgetown Law Review* 57 (1969).

Tancredi, Laurence R., ed. *Ethics of Health Care.* Washington, D.C.: Institute of Medicine, National Academy of Sciences, 1974.

Taylor, David. "Understanding the NHS in the 1980s." London: Office of Health Economics, 1984.

Taylor, Vincent. "How Much is Good Health Worth?" *Policy Sciences* 1 (1970).

Telfer, Elizabeth. "Justice, Welfare and Health Care." *Journal of Medical Ethics* 2 (September 1976).

Thomas, Lewis. *The Lives of a Cell.* New York: Viking Press, 1974.

Thurow, Lester. "Learning to Say 'No'." *New England Journal of Medicine* 311 (December 13, 1984).

_____. "Medicine vs. Economics." *New England Journal of Medicine* 313 (September 5, 1985).

Tocqueville, Alexis de. *Democracy in America.* 2 vol. Translated by Henry Reeve. New York: Schocken Books, 1961.

Townsend, Peter, and Nick Davidson. *Inequalities in Health.* London: Penguin, 1982.

Veatch, Robert M. "Voluntary Risks to Health: The Ethical Issues." *Journal of the American Medical Association* 243 (January 4, 1980).

_____. *A Theory of Medical Ethics.* New York: Basic Books, 1981.

_____. "A Novel Proposal." *Massachusetts Medicine* 4 (July/August 1986).

Veatch, Robert M., and Roy Branson. *Ethics and Health Policy.* Cambridge, Mass.: Ballinger, 1976.

Veatch, Robert M., and Morris F. Cohen. "The HMO Physician's Duty to Cut Costs." *Hastings Center Report* 15 (August 1985).

Vladek, B. C. "Medicare Hospital Payment by Diagnosis-Related Groups." *Annals of Internal Medicine* 100 (1984).

Waitzkin, Howard. "A Marxist View of Medical Care." *Annals of Internal Medicine* 89 (1978).

Walzer, Michael. *Spheres of Justice: A Defense of Pluralism and Equality.* New York: Basic Books, 1983.

Wessel, David. "Transplants Increase And So Do Disputes Over Who Pays Bills." *The Wall Street Journal* 73 (April 12, 1984).

Wickler, Daniel. "Persuasion and Coercion for Health: Ethical Issues in Government Efforts to Change Lifestyles." *Milbank Memorial Quarterly* 56 (1978).

Wildavsky, Aaron. "Doing Better and Feeling Worse: The Political Pathology of Public Health." In *Doing Better and Feeling Worse,* edited by John H. Knowles. New York: W. W. Norton, 1977.

Winslow, Gerald R. *Triage and Justice.* Berkeley, Calif.: University of California Press, 1982.

Wolff, Robert Paul. *The Poverty of Liberalism.* Boston: Beacon Press, 1968.

Index